'I'm [...]
I'm not y[...]
I know if you put these words into practice your life will change. Take a deep breath, decide on your first course of action, write it down, make it real and begin to plan out how to make it happen. The day you look back on where everything changed for you is about to begin.'

NOT ~~A~~ ~~LIFE~~ ~~COACH~~

NOT ~~A LIFE~~ ~~COACH~~

Push Your Boundaries.
Unlock Your Potential.
Redefine Your Life.

JAMES SMITH

HarperCollins*Publishers*

p.65 and p.106 Extracts from *Outliers* by Malcolm Gladwell. Copyright © 2008 published by Little, Brown and Company 2008, Allen Lane 2008, Penguin Books 2009. Reproduced by permission of Penguin Books Ltd.

p. 140 Extract from *The Story of Philosophy* by Will Durant. Reproduced by permission of SSA, a division of Simon & Schuster, Inc. Copyright © Will Durant, 1961.

p.155 Extract from *Sapiens* by Yuval Noah Harari. Copyright© 2015 by Yuval Noah Harari. Courtesy of HarperCollins Publishers.

p.157, p. 196 and p.208 Extracts from *The 4-Hour Workweek: Escape The 9-5, Live Anywhere, And Join The New Rich* by Timothy Ferriss. Copyright © 2007, 2009 by Carmenere One, LLC. Used by permission of Crown Books, an imprint of Random House, a division of Penguin Random House LLC. All rights reserved.

p.237 Extract from *Start With Why: How Great Leaders Inspire Everyone to Take Action* by Simon Sinek. Copyright © 2009 by Simon Sinek. Reproduced by permission of Penguin Books Ltd. © and by permission of Portfolio, an imprint of Penguin Publishing Group, a division of Penguin Random House LLC. All rights reserved.

While every effort has been made to trace the owners of copyright material reproduced herein and secure permissions, the publishers would like to apologise for any omissions and will be pleased to incorporate missing acknowledgements in any future edition of this book.

HarperCollins*Publishers*
1 London Bridge Street
London SE1 9GF

www.harpercollins.co.uk

First published by HarperCollins*Publishers* 2020

10 9 8 7 6 5 4 3 2 1

A catalogue record of this book is available from the British Library

HB ISBN 978-0-00-840484-0
TPB ISBN 978-0-00-840481-9

Printed and bound in Great Britain by
CPI Group (UK) Ltd, Croydon

Contents

PART III: FOUNDATIONS

PART IV: IDENTITY

PART V: COMFORT ZONES AND ESCAPISM

CONTENTS

Preface

If someone had asked me when I was twenty-one to write a book that could change lives, I wouldn't have considered myself able to change even one person's life for the better, or offer any advice of true value. But here we are, ten years on, and I've found myself doing exactly that – and doing it as a career. In a relatively short space of time, I have gained valuable perspective, experience and evidence that go beyond assumption and are void of unconscious bias, all to provide you with the opportunity to change the way you think. Let's put it this way: for the last decade, often without even realizing it, I've been preparing for this very moment, for you to pick up this book and read this very page.

In my first book, I delved into how to fix insecurities, physical issues and imbalance from the neck down; here, I look at all that exists from the neck up. I know what you are probably thinking right now: who the hell am I to give you advice? What puts me in a position of authority on these topics? I ask myself the same question most days, to be honest, and have thought to myself while writing each and every chapter: why should people listen to me?

I'm not trying to be an expert on life. I am not your leader, and I'm not asking you to follow me. I am not, nor can I be, irrefutably correct on every opinion I have. I am, like you and like everyone you know, only human.

The popular Greek proverb states that 'old men plant trees whose shade they know they shall never sit in'. When it comes to the art of true stoicism and many long-held discussions of philosophy, I often sit back and wonder whether it's all just a trail of people leaving advice they wish their younger selves could hear.

I wasted years of my life frustrated, deflated, disheartened and annoyed in the wrong job, chasing the wrong goals, eventually becoming the personal trainer that I wish had been there for me when I needed him. Now, I hope that I can be the coach I wish had been there when I was sleepwalking through my own life, held back by believing my own potential was limited.

Only you can take the reins of your own life and choose to make a change, but I can be the one to give you the tools to do so. This book is quite simply the book I wish had been there for me at crucial turning points of my life.

If you stop to look around and think about it, you will see there is an invisible blueprint to life that the majority of the world is following, and I can't help but think it's leaving so many people unfulfilled, unhappy and dissatisfied. Many seek and accomplish financial 'freedom', but it's to no avail when there is no sense of purpose. This book, I hope, will provoke necessary change; it will begin from the turn of the next page, but it won't finish with the turn of the last.

Where you'll be standing, who with, what you'll be doing and what you'll achieve are all going to be based on what you read and what you don't, who you keep in your life and those you let go. In the words of the author Charlie 'Tremendous' Jones: 'You will be the same person in five years as you are today except for the people you meet and the books you read.'

To leave chapters of this book unread will increase the chances that you will leave chapters of your life unlived and, without being unlocked, your potential could be limited, your growth stunted and your self-worth and everyday happiness could suffer.

PREFACE

This is not an ornament for your window ledge – it is not just a book *you plan to read*, a collation of motivating quotes or parables to live by; this is a lens through which to view the world, so that you can clearly see your underlying potential in the context of a spectrum that you couldn't see clearly before.

I am not your *life coach*. I am here with one sole purpose: to *change your life*.

So let's begin.

James

Introduction

What if I told you that by the time you finish this book perhaps nothing will have changed? Pretty uninspiring, right? You may be a few days older, maybe a few weeks. I don't know your reading speed or commitment to what I have to say. But ultimately things will be the same. Your phone will lose reception where it usually does, you'll still be daydreaming about that item of clothing you've been thinking about buying for the last few weeks and I expect you'll probably be using the same tube of toothpaste you are right now when you get to the end of this book. Riveting already, isn't it?

On a physical basis, you'll weigh about the same and have the same hairstyle. You'll also probably have the same job and day-to-day routine. And that very individual way you dry yourself with the towel when you get out the shower? All unchanged. However, these are not the metrics by which I want you to understand *change* if you commit to reading the next 275 pages. The changes I'm talking about could be so significant that you won't recognize the person you were just a short time ago. Not necessarily from the outside, maybe not even in the eyes of close family and friends, but in how you begin to realize and perceive certain things about your life.

Stop, take a look around, and you'll notice that everyone is climbing the ladder of life to see who can get to the highest rung. However, I don't see many people taking a moment to really think whether they're climbing the right ladder. It doesn't matter how high you climb it if, when you get to the top, you realize you've climbed the wrong one. It doesn't matter how fast you're going if you're not going in the right direction.

But if everyone else is doing it, how come I'm telling you you're wrong to do the same? Let's flip that for a second: am I saying you're wrong with your choices or am I alluding to the fact that your choices aren't 100 per cent right? And when I say 'right', I mean that if we were to sit down and look at what you want to do with your life and what you're currently doing with it, I think we could find some pretty blatant discrepancies. You'd probably offer excuses like, 'Now isn't a good time' or, 'If I had more financial freedom.' But I'm afraid the universe will not align with you and the seas will not part to create an easy path for you. That's life.

I've often said, 'If a million people believe something stupid, it's still stupid.' Humans are brilliant at telling themselves stories, like the elaborate ones about what happens when we die – some people are more concerned with the afterlife than their existing one. (That's not a dig at religion, but an example to consider in the wider context: if someone wanted you to buy shares, you'd want something tangible to back up their claims, wouldn't you? Just because someone else believes in it doesn't mean you should as well.)

I know what you're thinking – we're only human, right? Well, what does that even mean? Let's look at what being human is, because if there's one thing you need to know about human beings, it's that we're inherently dishonest. We lie and we can't help it. And this isn't exclusive to just us Homo sapiens, either. If we look across the animal kingdom, we can see it's prevalent among primates and all kinds of other species that barely resemble humans at all.

Not telling the truth isn't always a bad thing, though. Consider a knife, say: it's really about what you choose to do with it – you could harm someone or you could just butter their toast. Well, it's the same with a lie. And the reason I even mention this so early on in the book is this: you're feeding yourself lies – the harmful kind – on an ongoing basis, and that's not even the worst part of it, either. Want to know what's worse? You're believing them and therefore unaware of the harm they're causing, and it's having a profound impact on not just how you feel, but who you are and how you see yourself on a daily basis. Now, it's worth mentioning that harm in this context is deliberately inflicted by yourself on yourself; it's not a wound that's visible like a cut, but instead it is a set of limiting beliefs, poor values and the inability to back yourself to your full potential on days of the week that end in 'y'.

From this introduction to the last chapter of this book and everything in between you can become a completely transformed person with a new approach, mindset and entirely different beliefs to the person who is about to turn this page right now – but I need your full attention for just a handful of hours.

Now put this book down for a second, look around and tell me what you see. Most things you'll tend to see are governed by money, greed, quick hits of dopamine, instant gratification and calories. The problem with this is that we're *told* these things will make us happy. But I see money and calories as just the top of the list of currencies crippling the world's self-esteem.

Money, that's easy – you can buy the biggest yacht in the world, but one day you'll see a bigger one next to yours in the marina. There's a reason they say that the two best days of your life when you own a yacht are the day you buy it and the day you sell it. We're made to feel inadequate and that our lives should be governed by doing 'the right thing', such as buying a house or prioritizing how our CVs look, rather than travelling, taking risks or, most importantly, just enjoying it the best we can before the lights go out.

Then there are calories, hedonic foods, indulgences and gluttony for those who perhaps have issues like underlying unhappiness – that is why I wrote *Not a Diet Book*. I wanted to bring clarity to the concept of how all diets work the same way and that ultimately adherence and sustainability are at the nucleus of successful fat-loss regimes.

With this book I wanted to move away from calories and fitness and instead challenge your mindset, ethos and attitudes outside of that realm of your life to align you with a new way of thinking. Especially in the context of a largely nuanced and subjective word that, no matter what we say, we all crave and seek, sometimes without even knowing it: **success**.

Why is it that our younger, more adventurous, risk-taking inner child became so derailed from what they instinctively loved doing? Why have so many of us become dead set on seeing who can die with the most money? Why do we lie to ourselves about what we wish to accomplish or prioritize things in the way that we do? Why do we want people to follow us on social media, and take it so personally when they unfollow us? (Which, if you think about it, is merely to opt out of wanting to see what we're posting and sharing each day, hardly the stab in the gut it can feel like.)

We are so wrong about what success is, so many of us quite simply not being happy no matter what. We have more at our fingertips than we've ever had before, yet we struggle to feel happy about it. And we have days when we feel deflated and unmotivated despite the fact that, by comparison (which I'll come on to later), we have it so much better than others. Why?

Why do we quantify our self-worth with finances, materialistic purchases and how much it's possible to get laid, only to end up often overlooking the good life that has been in front of us the entire time?

And why are we blindly led to the blueprint for life by people who have spent a lifetime lying to themselves? It's like the blind leading the blind on how to pay taxes and then die.

The world becomes safer and an easier place in which to live. I know a lot of people don't believe this since COVID-19, but it's important to remember that couples used to, on average, have five to six children due to the fact that it was unlikely many would reach adulthood. Although (at the time of writing) there is an impending economic gloom for many, we still have access to doctors, antibiotics, state support and education. People think the world is getting worse, but it's getting better, I assure you. We've only had warm showers for around 150 years; no one even knew what a warm shower was before then. So, if you can be a pragmatist for a second, take your mind off the tabloid headlines and you'll see that the world continues to improve. Yet at the same time, the rates for people deciding to prematurely hit the eject button on their life continues to rise. Are we fucked or are we, perhaps, just idealizing the wrong things?

It worries me to see the number of people who are anxious, emotionally crippled, insecure and unhappy, while simultaneously being given the tools to mask their real feelings with a triple tap on a laughing-face emoji in the group chat. The systems in which we live, our methods of communication and what we're exposed to on social media all impact how we feel about ourselves, our place in the world, our purpose and our happiness. But are we truly broken or do we simply need to rethink our perceptions on elements of our lives that we have perceived incorrectly before?

I once thought I was lucky with my state of mental health. I even declared myself as someone who 'didn't suffer' with mental-health issues. I have since found that isn't the case at all; I was just much more proactive than I ever realized at protecting my state of mind, my 'mental wealth'. I am going to share a lot with you over the coming chapters about how you can protect yours too.

Let's say you're injured – do you know a physio? Toothache – you see a dentist. But do you know where to go when you're struggling with mental health – a person, a place or an organization that can help? Because you should. Athletes are proactive with avoiding injuries when possible, but they do happen; the same proactive approach should be taken with mental health – just like a check-up at the dentist. To spot things before they cause us too much pain. What could the possible negative implications be on proactively making contact with someone who could help you? You may not need them now, but in the future, it's better to have the person and not need them than vice versa. Look at the military, for instance – on standby at all times, usually at a cost of billions to taxpayers. An essential pre-emptive resource so that if things go bad, we're ready. If you're an athlete and your performance is of the utmost importance to you, it is worth getting even the slightest niggle looked at before it potentially gets worse. You'll come back from a muscle strain, but not everyone is coming back from their mental-health 'niggles', thus the importance of staying on top of mental health even before you think you might 'need' to.

But before we begin, let us be real with each other. This book can, if necessary, be read in a day. I know that; you know that. I'm asking for a day of your life (or maybe the evenings of one week or the lunch breaks of a fortnight), and in return, I am laying bare what could be the very notions to connect the dots in what will make you happier long-term.

You don't need a six-pack to be loved or taken seriously; you don't need to worry about how your CV looks to those who love you – or to a complete stranger, for that matter. You don't need to die with the most money in your bank account, because there are no shops in heaven. You just need to really understand success and happiness within the sphere of your own ambitions.

Objectively speaking, we need water, food, sunlight and somewhere to sleep each night to live our lives. But the rest of what we call 'life' is subjective; it's governed by our tastes, our feelings and our opinions. Don't forget that. Life is only influenced by your thoughts; your existing beliefs are tainted by a bullshit blueprint and it's time to rewrite your own. What's more, there are no rules to writing it, and when you do, you will experience empowerment like you've never felt before.

I know what you're thinking: I am happy, though. I am good, though.

What did I tell you about humans having that tendency to be dishonest? The worst bit is, I bet you even believe your thoughts that countered mine in the first place. But I'm not saying you're an unhappy person, just that you haven't even scratched the surface of your potential, self-determined success or happiness.

Right now, let me tell you this: **you're currently living in the part of your life you used to look forward to the most** and I bet you don't ever, for a second, give that enough thought to fully realize it, do you?

Social media drives self-esteem down, materialism up, self-worth into the floor and consumerism to the sky. You're a piece in someone else's board game and you don't realize it. You're not just lying to yourself but being lied to by society as a whole. People work too hard for money they don't need to buy non-essential things to impress people they don't like. The world remains full of people fucking exhausted and hungry in a bid to be in such good shape they could belong on the front cover of a magazine, while the bottom line is that … no one who truly matters really cares how much fat you're carrying as long as you're healthy, active and you have good banter. (I'm living proof of that.)

Imagine closing the last page of this book and realizing that not a lot has to change in your life, but a tremendous amount can change in your head. I am going to shake a metaphorical tree in many areas of your life; in some, you may clutch the branches so tight that you'll know I'm wrong, while in others you'll fall out of that tree and realize you were holding tight to a branch that wasn't the right one for you.

But either way, it's time for you and me to rewrite the norms and the rules to your existing beliefs, so we can align your journey with a destination that truly makes you happy and actually makes you feel successful. Not only that, but we can eradicate a lot of useless doubt, that constant feeling of undervaluing your ability, and we can stop you from getting in your own way so much. I am going to arm you with a new mindset and outlook so that you can begin adjusting anything that could potentially be wrong right now.

I hope I am wrong. I hope you're different. But I'm confident I'm not or I wouldn't have written this book. There are some very hard pills to swallow, but if you're ready for this, buckle up and let's begin.

PART I
ENVIRONMENT

The dictionary definition of environment is 'the surroundings or conditions in which a person, animal or plant lives or operates'. So, if a certain plant is thriving where it is, and we move it, the chances are very high that it will not survive, or it will take some time to adjust and recover. We can't label any environment as definitively good or bad, therefore it's subjective, and contextual. For instance, many things will die in a desert, but a cactus will thrive. A cactus is rather unique in its ability to store water, needing infrequent rainfall to maintain optimum internal conditions for survival. Now, this isn't called 'Not a Cactus Book', so I'll move on, but I just wanted to make the point that we should not automatically seek an objectively 'good' environment; we should seek the right one for our needs. What is a great environment for one plant could mean death for another and vice versa.

Animals are much the same as plants in this respect. For example, let's consider the temperature of water in which fishes* thrive and reproduce. One of the biggest issues with global warming is the effect it is having on our seas; ice on land is melting and when that ice makes its way into the sea it affects the salinity of the water, disrupting currents and fishes' habitats, leading to bigger environmental consequences. If it was up to a fish, we wouldn't be altering the

---

* I know for a second there you wanted to correct me and say the plural of fish is fish. It's actually a double plural and scientists who study fish will say 'fishes'. A few pages in and you're already becoming a smart arse.

environment in which they thrive, yet as humans we consistently choose to do so.

So, it's safe to say that our environment – or any environment – is crucial to thrive, to survive and, for us more consciously aware human beings, to be happy.

The Essentials

Strangely enough, our everyday human environment is not much of a conversation we have and it certainly doesn't gain much traction in discussions about what's truly important in our lives. Should you sit someone down and ask them what they'd like, they might say 'to win the lottery' (financial) or 'to go on a long holiday' (a break from existing job/routine). Rarely does anyone turn around and say, 'I'd like to live and exist in a better environment.' So many people land in an environment determined by a job, for example, as the first stepping stone, and then never leave it. The initial dull, dreary job may be a 'just-for-now' move, but before they know it, they're comfortable, and when challenged it's all too easy to say, 'I'll do it when I'm a bit older.'

Survival isn't that high on our agendas because we're all incredibly safe – statistically speaking, the safest yet since humans began on Earth. Of course you still need to look each way before crossing the road, get your vaccines and be sensible, but considering most people have running water, refrigerated food stores and electricity, I'd say that as far as an environment for survival is concerned, you're going to be just fine.

Where the environment really comes into play is with its connection to how much you enjoy it, therefore how happy it makes you. I'm not a hippie, but I do often refer to my 'soul' and what my soul would prefer. So, it's not my soul that wants pizza, but it is my soul that wants clear skies or to be near the sea. I've struggled for much of my life to understand this feeling properly. I would often just bury my urge for a different environment, believing the one I was in was the norm. And the norm only seemed that way because no one else was questioning it; not once did anyone around me say, 'Could I be happier somewhere else?' It's very important that we prioritize our environment over many other things; even the smallest change in metaphorical temperature can have a profound impact on your happiness. For instance, when you move in with someone – a partner, perhaps, or a new housemate – your job, salary, relationship with your parents, etc. all stay the same, but overnight your environment changes and many other aspects of your life with it, and it's not to be taken for granted.

The importance of change

Environment can be defined by physical factors such as country and climate. You can experience different environments by travelling and getting stuck in. I played rugby in New Zealand for six months. I got the offer to play through an agency online, and within three weeks I had quit my job, packed and flown to the other side of the planet on a whim. I learned that it wasn't my perfect environment, but it was an amazing perspective nevertheless. I worked on a farm, in forestry and even put up signs for a living. From sheep shearing to signage, I'd come a long way from wearing a suit, and even though I knew deep down that these jobs were not right for me, at least I wasn't bored. I found the change of environment very useful; it gave me experience and insight into different careers. People are so afraid to 'change lanes' in their profession, but just like dating, you sometimes need to play the field for essential perspective.

Other key factors to consider within your environment are the associated elements – for example, culture and who you spend time with are big factors. Hopefully you haven't forgotten that Charlie Tremendous Jones quote from earlier: 'You will be the same person in five years as you are today except for the people you meet and the books you read.'

What if I was to say that a huge number of the failures and successes you will face in the future are profoundly impacted by who you decide to spend time with in the coming years? Our environment is not just the bubble we live in, but the people within it as well. Many diets don't just fail because of a lack of willpower and temptation, but because of environmental factors and the people who surround the dieter. 'Go on, just one won't hurt,' from the unsupportive partner. 'Oh, but it's the weekend, relax!' We see this with relationships where perhaps there is a gap between the ambitions of each partner: 'It's the weekend, you shouldn't be working.' Or: 'It's getting late – put your laptop away.' The people you surround yourself with are either the wind in your sails or a headwind you're sailing against, and you must identify these. But don't grab your phone right away and begin the cull – not yet, anyway. Just keep it in mind. I always like to remind people that birds that fly in formation do so to reduce drag; you need the people by your side to be flying in your direction, and if they're not, it's not personal, but it's probably just not right. Those of you who read my first book may remember I opened with this quote:

> *Give me six hours to chop down a tree and I will spend the first four sharpening the axe.*
>
> Abraham Lincoln

Instead of wielding the axe straight away, you need to adopt a similar perspective to assembling your team for life, especially if your environment doesn't currently match your dreams. If you're not where you want to be, it's time to begin the process of moving closer to wherever that is, and you must identify who is with you and begin the painful job of recognizing who isn't. Humans copy each other, often subconsciously, in order to fit in. Take mirroring, for example: next time you're sitting with someone, cross your legs and wait to see how long it takes them to do the same. Then, shortly after, sit back and cross your arms, and see what happens. Humans, by their very nature, mirror each other. There is a fairly pseudoscientific communication known as NLP (neurolinguistic programming) where one of the tactics I've seen involves people copying other people's actions in a bid to promote a rapport, but I feel that some of these 'tactics' are rubbish. Watch someone yawn,* and you can't resist … someone has a giggling fit and you're suddenly laughing for no reason. Put all this together and you'll see the importance of who we surround ourselves with, as we're often connected to these people much more than we think. Personality also comes into play, with extroverts tending to mimic others more because being liked by

---

* Talking of yawns, some people believe yawning is to do with the brain cooling. Others draw direct parallels with empathy: 'The susceptibility to contagious yawning correlates with empathic skills in healthy humans.' (See References, p. 255.) For a long time, people have believed there's a connection between yawning and brain hypoxia (lack of oxygen), but this has been discarded since studies of people breathing air with mixed amounts of oxygen and carbon dioxide did not affect the participants' yawn rate. What's crazy to me is that yawning occurs in almost all vertebrates and has been spotted in foetuses at only twenty weeks. Interestingly, the studies on yawning are done on humans and chimpanzees and there is a spectrum from close friend to stranger, whereby the closer the person is to you, the more inclined they are to yawn. So next time you yawn and your partner or best friend doesn't, it may be a good time to reconsider the relationship … Just kidding. Yawning is one of many things that the world just doesn't know enough about to say for sure.

others is more important to them than it is to introverts. (See References, p. 255.)

So, coming back to the importance of what and who you surround yourself with, I want you to think of any time when you or someone you know has experienced tremendous success. Because it's often linked to change – not just any change, but change in environment, surroundings and the people who constitute your social and professional life. I'm not here to tell you how your environment needs to look or how it should be, just to ensure it's held high on your priority list and that you never take it for granted. The way we think about our environment and the choices we make about it can go a long way to explaining why some people feel broken and unmotivated. Didn't get that promotion? Didn't get invited to a party? Got rejected by a crush? Instead of spiralling into feelings of insecurity and a lack of self-worth, consider whether the environment you were trying to thrive in was the right one in the first place.

If we're not living to our fullest potential, I very much doubt it's *who* we are that's at fault as much as *where* we are and who we're associated with. So, whether your goal is fat loss, financial 'freedom' or just happiness and the feeling of being content with your work–life balance, putting a magnifying glass over your environment and those within it is crucial. Not everyone will survive, I warn you now; dead wood should be removed. Whether you're looking to get more from a business, a flowerbed or your immediate future, you must eliminate anything that does not serve a purpose in reaching your goals.

A strong associative environment* paired with an ideal physical one

---

* Associative environment is a term I've coined to talk about your environment in the context of who you associate with, not which country you're in or the weather.

is only going to produce an outcome of prosperity, happiness and the ability to thrive. Changing who you are takes time; changing who you surround yourself with and where you operate can be changed today.

'Wealth': Real Wealth Versus Money in the Bank

'If only I had more money ...' A huge misconception we often feed ourselves is that if we had more money, we'd have more happiness. But I am afraid it's bullshit. Likewise, we know, sadly, that having a good credit rating or a trust fund won't protect us from mental or physical health issues. It doesn't matter how much we're worth – if we don't value the right things, money won't buy us out of feeling unhappy. Let me introduce you to a concept known as income satiation.

Income satiation

Does happiness rise indefinitely with income, or is there a point at which higher incomes no longer lead to greater wellbeing?

Interestingly, in the literature I've looked at, I have found the threshold seems to be around £60,000 (110,000 AU$), beyond which increases in income no longer improve people's ability to do what matters most to their emotional wellbeing, such as spending time with people they like and enjoying leisure. We seem to think of money and pleasure as being on a linear* scale – more money = more happiness – and I think that's why, all too often, we envy the richest amongst us. (See References, p. 255.)

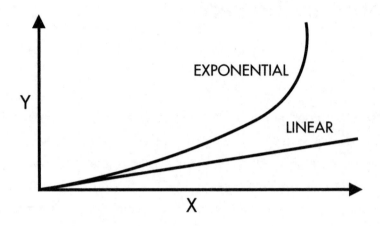

Now, this isn't to say that if you're not earning a certain amount you can't be happy, quite the opposite. But it is to explain the diminishing returns after a certain point.† By eradicating the notion of a linear route to happiness we can begin to understand that's not how we work and it's not how the world works either.

'When income rises beyond this value, the increased ability to purchase positive experiences is balanced, on average, by some negative effects. A recent psychological study using priming methods provided suggestive evidence of a possible association between high income and a reduced ability to savour small pleasures.' (See References, p. 255.)

---

* Linear is a straight line plotted across a graph, whereas exponential growth would usually have an upward curve.

† I don't want to get caught up in the numbers here, as I know incomes vary hugely, but the findings of the various studies and the meanings behind them are applicable and crucial to all of us.

It's very interesting to see that when people were reminded about their wealth they then spent less time savouring a piece of chocolate. Sounds weird, right? It was reported that these people also exhibited reduced levels of enjoyment compared with participants not reminded of wealth. This is some of the evidence that supports the notion that having easy access to the 'best things' in life could very well be your Achilles' heel, preventing you from savouring, enjoying and making the most of the little things. More is not always better; happiness, fulfilment and quality of life are not to be considered linear on paper.

I was invited as a guest to fly to Amsterdam on a private jet a few years ago. The jet was, quite frankly, ridiculous, with sofas to relax on and never-ending quantities of champagne served, and throughout the flight I had one feeling I couldn't shake: the notion of how much the experience was going to ruin normal air travel in the future. (We flew back from Amsterdam on an EasyJet flight – quite the contrast, I can tell you.) When I was a child, sitting on any plane was an adventure that would keep me awake with excitement the night before. Now, nothing had changed except what I had been exposed to. The point I want to make is that I very much doubt regular private-jet users can experience even business-class flights without feeling cramped. If you reach a certain level of wealth, one person's dream (such as flying busi-ness class) can be someone else's idea of travelling like cattle.

I don't think many of us always realize that wherever we sit on the scale of earnings, markers for happiness remain very much the same – love is the same and even feeling content with your day is the same. I want you to think about that: if you earned half of what you do currently, you could still be just as happy; and if you earned ten times as much, the same applies – the only thing that changes is your spending habits. To put it simply – expending all of your energy on thinking about how you can earn more money is not a wise investment of your time or effort. Coming home and getting into comfortable clothes, sitting back with a glass of wine or a beer and putting your feet up on the table? That feeling is the same, no matter where you do it.

Corporate life and the 'herd instinct'

Moving on, the next terrible misconception we are all so often guilty of is the assumption, or even belief, that 'I'll do that when I'm older'.

Rewind the best part of seven years and you'll find out about the time I spent six months backpacking in Southeast Asia. Of course I did – I was a typical twenty-something from Berkshire, unsure of which direction to take in my life. But before I tell you about my first happy-ending massage (which was great) let me tell you about the 'the herd instinct' and how it affected me as an adult, ready to take on the world.

When the time came to enter the 'world of work' (remember that blueprint I told you about?), I applied for a job in the corporate world because, to me, I suppose in hindsight, it was the only logical pathway to that elusive six-figure salary. I put on my cheap suit, shiny black shoes and learned how to tie a tie. Why? Because it was what 'everyone else' was doing when they got to my stage in life.

Now, wearing a suit has no functional purpose beyond having more pockets than casual attire. I never once questioned why I was doing it or whether the money I'd be paid for the hours in my office cubicle would be worth it. I simply thought to myself: how else can I make my parents proud, buy a house and get a nice car without such a salary? I love cars, and from when I was a teenager to my mid-twenties they got faster, more luxurious and newer, but at the time of writing, I haven't had a car in years and only ride my trusted cruiser skateboard around. I hope you believe me when I tell you it makes me far happier than any car ever did.

The six-figure salary to me seemed like the only logical stepping stone – not once did I ever think my values were misaligned, just that I needed new shoes and to shave for the interview and pretend I cared about it a lot more than I really did. So, I held my glass of water in my shaking hand (it kept my palm cool and reduced the clamminess that was a frequent occurrence in this type of interview). Then I took a sip of water as my interviewer got to the end of his sentence, which bought me another couple of seconds to conjure a good response without seeming like I was thinking too much. All tricks of the trade, like an illusionist, my only care being getting the job so I'd have money in my bank account come the end of the month.

Well, the cool-palm/water-sipping trick paid off because I got that job. And most others I interviewed for.

There was a weird moment when I sat at my desk on my first day in that job, adjusted my chair and ensured my monitor was at the right height so that I didn't get a neck problem (given the huge amount of time I'd be staring at it, week on week). I looked at my phone and I thought to myself: this is it. You think of your payslip, how much it means per month after tax and what that can do for those around you. You think about 'career opportunities', 'progressions' and 'incentives'. You line up your mobile phone in a perpendicular manner to the keyboard and think of the lovely arrangement you have in front of you.

I found this mindset of thinking down, not up. What I mean is that I remember my salary was around £20,000 (36,400 AU$) – I thought to myself: OK, that's £1,600 (2,900 AU$) a month and about £1,200 (2,185 AU$) after tax. I then divided it by the hours in a nine-to-five job, and thought that's £7.50 (13.65 AU$) an hour, comparing it to what I earned in the pub, which was £6 (11 AU$) an hour. Then, if they 'match' your pension contribution, you feel like you're getting free money (although I'm pretty sure that when you do the maths it's not as glamorous as you think) – for some this kind of security may be what they crave, but is trading the best years of your life for a future pension that covers a much smaller proportion of your life really a good marker of contentment? The tiny increase of £1.50 (2.70 AU$) an hour made me feel accomplished at the time, but there was one key difference: I had actually enjoyed working in the pub.

So, I'd found myself doing something I never really wanted to do, what seemed like **the right thing to do**, only because everyone else was doing it. I was following the herd. They all seemed happy, so I told myself what I now know is one of many lies I've told myself over the years: that I was happy working in that corporate world, soon to be consumed by the rat race.

The 'herd instinct' goes hand in hand with that blueprint I keep referring to, which so many of us follow by default. Why do we not challenge the status quo? Why is it perfectly acceptable to do something you don't enjoy so that you can live for the weekend? You'll get carried away Friday and Saturday, only to spend Sunday miserable in bed, half dreading work the next day, while the other half is suffering from the hangover. I like to remind people that Mondays do not suck. If you feel that way, it's not Mondays that are the problem, but the current structure and routine in your life.

So, there I was, fresh-faced, new to the corporate way of living, and in the office on day one, I was initially tested by making the tea for those around me. Do you know what I decided to do? I made the worst tea I possibly could to ensure I wasn't asked to do it again. In hindsight, intentionally making terrible tea could legitimately rank as the highlight of my dull, dreary days in the corporate world. I developed another trick, due to the rigidity of the hours and only being able to leave for home at 5.30 p.m. (it always annoyed me that regardless of how hard I worked, I'd still have to hit the same arbitrary amount of outward calls and have to leave at the same time each day): I'd often ask who wanted a cup of tea at 5.15 p.m. (no one, obviously, as it was almost time to go), then leave the office via a fire escape, out of sight of most of my colleagues. If my managers asked where I was come 5.25, everyone would say I was making a cup of tea, unknowingly covering my back.

Being exposed to the corporate world – people in higher positions than me, earning more money than me, having nicer things than I had … You wake up, you go to work, you come home and you try to enjoy the finite period of time between that and when you go to sleep. Is it any wonder that over the years I became fixated on my job title (which changed weekly when I was bored on LinkedIn), my income and the materialistic things everyone else had? Take a suit, for instance. I fucking hated wearing a suit, but within months I was thinking about how I needed a nicer one, a better fit, more expensive. I wanted a more expensive version of something I didn't even want, to impress people I didn't actually even like who earned more money than I did.

This all came to an end when I snapped. When I just couldn't do it any more. I needed to hit pause on life and just escape for a bit. So, I sold my fancy car and flew to Southeast Asia. Time slowed down for me then. I spent some days just worrying about how many beers I was going to have and others about what books I should read. I'd admire how some of the locals had what appeared to be so little, yet they had a sense of happiness much greater than anyone else's back home – even those with the six-figure salaries.

For me, in hindsight, I am so grateful I snapped when I did. It taught me a lesson about who I was, what I stood for, what I was willing to do and what I wasn't. I don't mean to completely shit on the corporate world, but in my experience, it's where I found that most organizations trade as much of your time and effort as they can for the least amount of money you'll accept to do it. Read that again: every salary is quite literally the least amount of money someone is willing to pay you for your finite amount of time on this planet.

It's not all grim, however. There are 'incentives', rewards like an Amazon voucher for picking up the phone enough times each day; and they'll even let you wear jeans to work on a Friday to make you feel like you're getting something out of the deal, too. Most people within the corporate world have to work to something called 'KPIs', which stands for key performance indicators. Although they're presented as a way to keep track of performance, they are largely to make sure you're doing enough; when someone isn't motivated to do a task, KPIs are a good way to ensure it gets done anyway. And if that doesn't hit home for many readers, what about this nugget here: not only do you get a pretty shit deal, you also, in most cases, sign a contract to let an organization design almost all aspects of your life for you.

These organizations, more often than not, decide when you wake up, when you eat, when you go home and (to them), most importantly, what you earn for your 'work'. I say 'work' in inverted commas because it's human nature to stretch whatever task is at hand across the amount of time you allocate to it. I'll expand on this later in the book, but many hours in the 9–5 are not spent working; they're just spent staring at a computer screen bored and worrying that you need to look busy.

When someone asks you why you're in that job, because you can't conjure up anything more compelling you'll immediately jump to the 'perks' and 'benefits' you get with the role: free dental, 5 per cent pension matched and £20 (36 AU$) contribution to your gym membership each month. In exchange for enduring busy public transport, sitting in traffic, wearing a suit on the hottest day of the year and becoming an expert in appearing to look busy every day.

I wish there was another word to describe it, but I felt very suffocated by the structures in place when I was in the corporate world. Now, I know that it suits some people, but for me I couldn't thrive in those surroundings. It's not that I was broken, but **the environment wasn't right for who I was**. My advice to others would be to really gauge if you're working in an environment that is right for you; just because it's right for everyone else doesn't mean it's going to be a good fit for you. For example, I have always spoken about dieting being like a tailored jacket: it needs to be thrown on and tailored to the person over time; what might fit one person perfectly may be an awful fit on someone else. And we need to take the same pragmatic approach to our work environments and to realize that we're not broken or outcasts if it doesn't fit – we're just sometimes in the wrong place. No harm in that, just something to be aware of. Because enduring something that isn't right only makes it worse over time, not better.

There's a parable I love to think about whenever I need to remind myself of the important things in life. It's about a fisherman and a businessman.

THE FISHERMAN AND THE BUSINESSMAN*

A successful businessman on vacation was at the pier of a small coastal village when a small boat with just one fisherman docked alongside him. Inside the small boat were several large yellowfin tuna. The businessman complimented the fisherman on the quality of his fish and asked how long it took to catch them.

The fisherman proudly replied, 'Every morning, I go out in my boat for thirty minutes to fish. I'm the best fisherman in the village.'

The businessman, perplexed, then asked, 'If you're the best, why don't you stay out longer and catch more fish? What do you do the rest of the day?'

The fisherman replied, 'I sleep late, fish a little, play with my children, spend quality time with my wife and every evening we stroll into the village to drink wine and play guitar with our friends. I have a full and happy life.'

The businessman scoffed. 'I am a successful CEO and have a talent for spotting business opportunities. I can help you be more successful. You should spend more time fishing and with the proceeds, buy a bigger boat. With the proceeds from the bigger boat, you could buy several boats and eventually, you would have a fleet of fishing boats with many fishermen. Instead of selling your catch to just your friends, you can scale up to sell fish to thousands. You could leave this small coastal fishing village and move to the big city, where you can oversee your growing empire.'

The fisherman asked, 'But how long will all this take?'

* Unknown source

To which the businessman replied, 'Fifteen to twenty years.'

'But what then?' asked the fisherman.

The businessman laughed and said, 'That's the best part. When the time was right, you would announce an IPO and sell your company stock to the public and become very rich. You would make millions!'

'Millions – then what?'

The businessman went on, 'Then you would retire. Move to a small coastal fishing village where you would sleep late, fish a little, play with your kids, spend time with your wife, stroll to the village in the evenings where you could sip wine and play guitar with your friends.'

Why does the plan for everyone have to revolve around accomplishing so much only to then go back to doing not a lot at all? The fisherman had his own values and it's rare to see that these days. Everyone else blindly has the mindset of the businessman. To give everyone the same blueprint to follow in life or to aspire to is just like giving them all the same thing to eat each day. It overlooks the simple fact that we're all hugely different and that we all want and need different things to be happy and truly succeed. **My closing thought for this section is this: out of the businessman and the fisherman, who is truly the wealthiest when it comes to life?**

Communication: How to Talk to Yourself and Others

Communication is such an important element of all human behaviour and relationships. Even the slightest improvements in communications can add profound benefits to your life.

Social Media 101: Who's your audience?

For my social-media presence to grow I had to forge an identity, a brand, within a particular environment – online. I would have to tailor this brand to the social-media platform, the person I had in mind and how I would communicate with them. One of the most interesting things from a marketing and social-media perspective is being incredibly clear on your 'avatar'. Who you're speaking to and how you speak to them. You may notice on TV, when you listen to car adverts, for instance, the voice on the advert has the exact person who is buying the car in mind. A pick-up truck or a van will be in a male voice with a working-class tone. For something a bit more high-end, you'll note a more 'well-spoken' voice. Many personal trainers make the mistake of communicating with other personal trainers on social media, therefore targeting the wrong audience and using the wrong language. You must know who you are talking to in order to get them to listen, and that applies to all aspects of life, not just social media.

The language and how you put across the information needs to be right.

Instagram, for me, is a more crass and punchy forum, while Facebook is a little slower-paced due to the nature of videos being in a longer format, and my podcast is an opportunity to have a conversation that can last hours opposed to seconds; I don't need to edit out any pauses in what I say and I can have someone's attention for their entire commute. Podcast James is like I am sitting in their passenger seat, while Instagram James is like I just got in the elevator with them and I'm getting out on a different floor.

This is not a way of being dishonest or tricking people; it's merely about being the right chameleon colour for the environment I am in at the time. On Instagram I might only have three seconds to capture someone's attention before they scroll past, ignore me, swipe away, go to another app or even unfollow me because I'm not entertaining them enough. I'm lucky on a good day if 5–10 per cent of my following see any given post, let alone interact with it. There's an art to social media that many don't see. You're talking to someone in a very crowded room, and you only have so long to impress, get your point across and get out with contact information.

The problem with finite thinking: how to ~~win~~ social media

The biggest thing that people get wrong with social media is thinking that they can win at it. I'm sorry but you can't win at it, but again, you can't lose at it either.

No post or video I publish can technically fail. **It's only a failure if I have the wrong metrics or values surrounding its success in the first**

place. If I base its success around arbitrary likes or views, it could 'fail', but that's the wrong way to see it. You can't sit in the fancy part of a plane with the amount of likes or double taps your last post got – that's how you set yourself up for the false notion of being able to fail social media. Social media serves a purpose, but it's often misconstrued by so many. To me, I see it very much like giving out flyers in an area to build a business: the more doors the better, and I expect most of them will go unnoticed. If a modern-day flyer campaign had a 1 per cent success rate, they'd be very happy with the outcome. When you can get your outlook into the marketer's mindset that a 99 per cent failure rate is completely fine, as long as you deliver to enough doors, you not only become mentally invincible and robust, but incredibly successful in your line of work.

Each day I set myself **my own** values and metrics. My outcome for success is posting content that will help people, realign their train of thought and be of benefit to the majority of those who see it. No number of likes, shares or comments can detract from my personal values for success with each post. With that, of course, I then at times collect data from people in the form of email addresses. I see the social-media posts like little jabs, then when you set yourself up with a right hook you can ask for someone's contact details to then try to sell to them further down the line. I like to utilize the law of reciprocity when I do this:* if I give enough to them, they'll hopefully feel inclined to give back with something which can seem so trivial like an email address.

People misunderstand social media and what it actually does. It's a means of getting in front of people and that's about it. People assume that Instagram or Facebook pay you the more followers you have. They

---

* Law of reciprocity: when someone does something nice for you, you will have a deep-rooted psychological urge to do something nice in return.

don't. Most people give up on social media because they haven't even realized what they should want from it. For me, simply, I just need email addresses. My years of pursuit of those emails grew my following as a by-product; just growing your followers doesn't do anything to your business bank account. That's why washed-up celebrities would literally promote poison in a bottle for a payslip; they have the following, but not enough business brains to monetize it in an ethical way. No one would care if I had 10 million email addresses, but they do care if I have a million followers. The first is actually much more powerful, but society just has generally different values about the metrics across the board and many naively follow the herd's idea of social-media success. Therefore, many are left unfulfilled from their efforts.

Life, relationships and business are not purely transactional. You need three key things to conduct a business: people need to **know you**, **like you** and **trust you**. Without all three you have nothing as a brand or business. I feel that no matter what I post about or talk about, if it plays into those three things, I am doing all right. Social media is not a popularity contest for anyone. We should all know we cannot please everyone.

Each day on social media I can achieve my own goals and win in that sense, but you can't actually win at social media itself. So utilizing social media in a bid to see who has the largest penis or biggest following is, in some way, simply setting yourself up to fail. When I see language like 'THE MOST' or 'THE BEST' I can straight away spot the mindset of finite thinking. It's the polar opposite of the long-game attitude to life. I don't want to have THE BEST business or be the BEST jiu jitsu athlete in the world; it's stupid to even say. However, I want to grow my business over time and develop my skills whenever I can. See how even the language used separates a goal from the long game and short game. I'll clarify further:

There are things in life that are finite and those that are infinite, by which I mean some things can be won and others can't. For instance, a game of rugby has a beginning, a half-time and a final whistle to end the game; there are rules laid out and the game can be won or lost. **It's a finite game**. However, in the games of business, life, finances or social media (or even love), you cannot win – it's infinite, and the best part is that there are no rules.

Thinking of some of the most successful and most brilliant minds of our time – Bill Gates, Warren Buffett, Oprah Winfrey, Steve Jobs – I don't believe any of them would have aimed for short, finite wins to see who could have the most of something. Instead, I think they had a long-game mentality, not to winning per se, but perhaps changing the status quo or the way people see things currently. Whether it was the most innovative technology or running a business to provide solutions to people's problems, I doubt they'd get caught up with who sold the most computers or made the most money in the second quarter of 2014.

The mission statements of Amazon and Google never reflected finite thinking:

Amazon: 'Earth's most customer-centric company.'

Google: 'To organize the world's information and make it universally accessible and useful.'

Neither of them set out to be a billion-dollar business. That's a finite approach.

TASK

If you're passionate about something, why don't you write about it? Why not set up a social-media page for it? I personally find it therapeutic to post each day, and you don't need to get caught up with how many followers your page has either, nor the likes. That's just you subconsciously quantifying the success, value, performance and worth of your page based solely on the herd instinct of the many who have come before you with poorer values than those you currently hold. So what if it doesn't have millions of followers, if it makes you feel good and serves a purpose? Who the hell can say otherwise?

Fall in love with the process and see what happens; you may monetize in a few years, you may not. There are no rules. Remember, social media and your therapeutic posting are not a finite game; there is to be no winner, nor is it about seeing who has 'the most'. If posting about your passion brings you a bit of pleasure, then you're winning already. Many don't experience that in life. If you enjoy making wooden tables, then make them and find a local marketplace online to sell them. Who doesn't need a custom-made table in their house? You can align what you love with making a living. Or just do it for fun. I don't care how much you do or don't earn from it. Just do me a favour and fucking do it.

So many people around me in my line of work fall into the trap of seeing who can die with the most followers or who can get the most likes on their social-media posts. By doing so not only are most people setting themselves up to fail, but they have their values for what **real**

success is largely wrong, and I feel that there is not genuine happiness to be found with these poor values.

Social media for me started out as a place to post helpful articles to reduce the amount of time I spent getting rejected on the gym floor. However, it very quickly evolved into a marketplace where I could share content to help people. If I am honest with you, it was also a place to challenge my fears. For years, and still to this day, I've been petrified of being wrong (or being persecuted for being wrong) and being outed as a fraud and a charlatan. That fear doesn't go away. It's constantly there. But you can't always talk about it because the people who need your help need it to be delivered in an authoritative manner. To doubt yourself all the time is to do a disservice to those who need your assistance in the first place.

I have a fierce rivalry with another man in a similar profession to mine. Over the last few years, people have gone so far as to insinuate that there's hatred or animosity between us. I emailed the person in question a few years ago (and I'm sure he'd remember it) simply to let him know that in the world we live in, we punch up, not down and not to take it personally. The sentiment that 'you never get put down by people above you in life' has helped me deal with my own fear of failure and the rebuttal that usually comes hand in hand with it.

I strangely have so much to thank social media for. Not just because it enabled me to become a bestselling author or to operate a large online business, but because it put me on a track to discover the single most important thing that makes me happy on a daily basis, which no one and nothing can take from me. I learned something about who I am and what makes me happy, and it can all be summed up in five simple words I discovered via a book called *Mindset* by Carol Dweck:

Becoming is better than being.

Through the pursuit of my own values on social media, it finally made sense to me. My early content was pretty awful, and to be honest, I wouldn't have it any other way. Since I am just honing the skill over time, I do it outside of social media with talks, writing books and many other things, especially Brazilian jiu jitsu, which is the single best sport I have ever discovered or taken part in, and which I will talk about later in the book.

There is no finite end point to all of this. To think there is sets us up to fail from the get-go. Each and every day to me is about doing it a little better than I did before. **My trajectory is far more important than where I currently am.** When I was a personal trainer sitting in a café writing articles for free, all I wanted to do the following day was write a better article. It was therapeutic. I enjoyed putting on my head-phones, zoning out from the world and just typing away, knowing deep down there was satisfaction to the point that if just one person read it I could change their perspective without ever having met them.

Fast forward a handful of years and all I care about is that my second book helps more people than the first and that my second TED Talk can impact more people than the first. It's the same process, it's just shuffled up a notch since that first article back in the day that only thirteen people viewed. Without social media I am not sure I would have found myself on this path, so for that I am grateful, and for every perceived negative associated with it I think there are positives that are not often weighed up.

Social media helped to detach me from the blueprint completely and I forged my own rule set in what is a very new way of operating a business and a brand – through a smartphone, tablet or computer.

There is no finite number of followers I desire, no financial situation I dream about, no yacht I want to buy and no set standard of content or writing I produce. **As long as I try my hardest to incrementally**

improve, I am happy. That's what I've discovered makes me happy. Sure, I've seen some impressive payslips in my time, but they can't compare to a simple comment on a post that says, 'That's your best post yet, James.' There is an insight into my thinking and values, whereby what I post is held in higher regard than what I earn. And that's good values in a nutshell.

I was asked by a close friend how I felt about writing 'book two', as I named it during the writing process. And I honestly took so much satisfaction from the process itself that I said to my friend, 'I am happy.' Nothing on top of that could make me happier. Writing this book, knowing someone would read it, makes me much happier than any sale or royalty I make from it. If you see me on my book tour, I'll be ecstatic – not from book sales, but from sharing a space with my best friends and the people who bought my book. That feeling and emotion can't be put in a bank account or quantified in sales figures. As long as I feel like my ability to write a better book has improved, I've won before the first sale ever occurs.

Understanding your own mindset

Carol Dweck has helped me identify two types of mindset: growth vs fixed. The fixed mindset gets very caught up with what has happened and thinks the worst; they think they're a failure if things don't go as planned. The growth mindset thinks about what they can do to improve their situation, even just a fraction, so that next time they can hopefully do better. **What I find personally is that the biggest differentiator between growth and fixed mindsets is how open you are to learning:**

A growth mindset is defined as a belief that construes
intelligence as malleable and improvable.

Carol Dweck (See References, p. 255.)

For instance, if you're not willing to learn, and you believe you can't become better or smarter, you think: what's the point in reading a book? Those who are willing to learn, willing to read and willing to study don't just think it, they *know* that through that book there's a chance they can become a slightly smarter version of themselves. And the best bit about those with a growth mindset is that if they finish the entire book and learned nothing, they can at least sit back and be happy with the fact that the book they just finished was probably not the right book for them.

If you take one thing from my book right here, it's that if you can just become more willing to learn, there can be an overnight shift in mindset that will allow you to become someone who is more of the growth mindset and less of the fixed. One of the most powerful tools for achieving a strong growth mindset is to realize that you can overcome anything that life throws at you. And if you can't do that right now, in time you can, if you're willing to put the work in. You can see any obstacle as a challenge.

Think about how many changes you have experienced in the last few years: your watch, phone, haircut, trainers or maybe even a house or car. But how many people in the space of even a decade have a change in mindset? Sometimes the most powerful and most needed change can occur somewhere you didn't even expect – not on your wrist or on your feet, but inside your head.

Failure is the condiment that gives success its flavour.

Truman Capote

Dwelling on past experiences or failures is of no use to us. Every failure is a blessing and the past is really the foundation that supports you in the present. **Mistakes are imperative and to be seen as adjustments necessary for the right direction. The good isn't the good without the bad.** Instead of focusing on what happened before, we must put all our mental energy into what is ahead, readying ourselves for the next hurdle, the next failure. **How we react to adversity is much more important than the adversity itself.** Embrace it, look forward to it; without failure ahead the future would seem much more bleak, possibly even boring. Therefore, future failures are something to look forward to, to cherish and to face with gratitude, not despair.

We also can't dwell on things that haven't happened. Worrying about something from your past and how it may crop up in the future. Instead of worrying about it, just think about how you can own it. You may have done something stupid when you were younger, but everyone does. I sometimes sit back and worry about whether or not I sent anyone a dick pic as a drunk teenager, but thinking about that is only going to drain me, so why worry? Why open the door to anything that's going to drain my energy for no positive return? We like to think of ourselves as one person, but the truth is we're many different versions of ourselves, as over the years we grow with experience and we develop knowledge. The person we are later in life perhaps wouldn't do what the younger version did. That doesn't make us bad, though; it just means we've changed and that shouldn't warrant any type of anxiety. If it happens, you will deal with it. **Don't worry about the speed bumps in the road until you see one that's worth slowing down for.**

If I look back at my biggest failures, they are the aspects of my life I am most grateful for. If you think about yours, I am sure you would agree. I don't need much from you right now – just that you cherish

33

the next hurdle instead of worrying about it. Time spent worrying is time wasted, let me tell you that for free.

So it's not just who we are, it's not just what we do; it's not just what is going to happen and it's not just dwelling on what has happened. Sometimes we need to sit and think about where we are right now and who we are surrounding ourselves with, to allow us to consider whether we need to adjust these things for long-term positive change. If you want a tree to grow to its full potential, you'd best think carefully about where you plant it.

PART II
VALUES

A value isn't just how much something costs; it's an integral part of our persona and identity. It signifies what we determine as being important in life, it's how we decide what we want, yet so many of us lose sight of our values. Our values are reflected in how we behave each and every day, so I hope that I can help you to rediscover what they are and ensure you pay greater attention to them.

Values of Success: So, What If It All Goes Wrong?

When I was twenty-eight, I had what I can only call 'a moment'. During this period of my life, I was experiencing what many would call relative 'success'. I'd get high fives walking down the beach in Sydney and requests for selfies on nights out from people who watched my content. Considering that for 90 per cent of my life up until writing this book that had never happened before, it was hugely overwhelming. You see, when people see you have a big social media following, they paint a picture of your life, and there's often not a lot of regard for how new it is for you. For a stranger to know so much about you or feel like they know you already is a phenomenon unique to the age of social media, and although I have so much gratitude for it, it's also kind of weird. Brilliantly weird, but weird. However, before getting into the social science of social media I want to tell you about a time when I was sitting in a steak restaurant in Sydney.

It was a summer's evening and I was with friends. I ordered my steak and had a little moment when I just looked around and took in my surroundings. It was a nice, normal evening. People were happy, the sun was setting and I was with good friends. I sat there and thought to myself: do you know what? If nothing works out, I'll just work here in this steak restaurant. I'll work the 4-or-5-p.m.-until-close shift, I'll do it five or six nights a week. During the day, I'll go the beach, I'll learn to surf and I'll get a dog. I'll give the dog my attention all day. I'll walk him and tie him up in a nice spot when I surf and then go home to nap or tan before my evening shift.

This isn't to say that we can all work in a restaurant as an easy way out of chasing our ambitions, but instead that 'success' can be found in places other people may not see from the outside. And that's fine too, because **success is internal and not a value we should chase to please other people**.

A simple job that isn't stressful may not make you the best-paid person in your friendship group, but it could make you a better friend, a better student in your hobby and even a more attentive lover. **We must always refer back to the metrics of success and remove our egos from any idea of the good life.** The restaurant wasn't an ambition, but more of a fail-safe that made me feel more confident to take risks.

Since that 'moment' over the medium-rare steak I have taken up Brazilian jiu jitsu and I will continue to devote myself to being a student of the sport until I physically can't do it any more. I am well aware that I'll never be considered successful in it to the outside world; I mean, think about it – realistically, I am just not going to be a superstar jiu jitsu athlete. That doesn't mean that it can't make me happy every single day, though (plus, that's only about success to the outside world). To me, the feat of just obtaining my next belt promotion could be enough, as **I set my own metrics for success**. For someone else, it could be different; it could just be turning up to three sessions a week. Only if I compare myself to the best competitors in the world can I be left feeling deflated. Do you see the correlation with our work life now? I'll talk about the humility that the sport has given me later on in the book, but for now, understand that between someone who does the sport as a hobby and someone else who competes and wins at the highest level, both can experience tremendous success based on their own metrics and values of what that means to them – and no one can take that away from them.

I want you to consider this, too. I could win a competition at blue belt in the next year. That could easily make me just as happy as someone else would be winning the worldwide black belt title. What I want you to realize is that the level of happiness we'd feel could, and most likely would, be exactly the same. Where the level of accomplishment sits on the scale doesn't influence the amount of happiness you get from it. What if I told you that I was just as happy from two very different victories: the first was when a man sat next to me in a café in the UK five years ago. This man paused, looked at me and said, 'I like reading your blogs.' To me, that was huge; although it was only a mile from the gym I was working in and in the very café in which I wrote them I could not believe my luck. The second was the recognition in becoming a *Sunday Times* bestselling author. But it felt the same. The scale of the victories, objectively speaking, is substantially different; but how they felt to me was the same. **You do not need to be the best in the world to be happy, as long as you choose the level you want to be happy at.**

I feel that in the world we live in we're made to feel that we must be in spectacular professions in order to be happy with them. But we don't. It's a bit like being an 'on paper' average athlete: as long as you're happy doing it, then who can say different? I used to date a Norwegian girl, and I'll never forget a conversation I once had with her dad. (He only said two things to me for the entire year and a bit that I dated his daughter.) We were out food shopping, and there was a lad, a good-looking lad, sat at the checkout of what, truth be told, was a bit of a shithole of a supermarket. The lad spoke fantastic English and had good banter (I'm pretty sure he made me laugh with an inside joke only British people would understand).

As we got out to the car park I said, 'I can't understand what a good-looking lad is doing in a job like that. How is he not doing something better – better paid or more interesting?'

And her dad turned to me and said, 'Well, James, some people behind closed doors have very complicated lives and therefore require very simple jobs.'

I'd never thought about it like that. And I've never forgotten it either. The second thing he told me was: 'All Norwegians are born with skis on their feet. Some, however, decide when they grow up to take them off.' That made me feel a lot better – partly about how terrible I was at skiing, but that wasn't quite his point. (In fact, I may have to tap him up for some more nuggets in this book as we go on.) I think his point (which means more to me the more I think about it) was that in life we are all born with everything we need to accomplish anything, but along the way, some of us, for whatever reason, feel the need to remove our skis, to throw in the towel and no longer pursue what we set out to do. Anyone who has ever gone skiing will testify to two things: in most cases, especially when you start out, those skis will come off; however, just as easily, they click back on. And that's not influenced by how long they have been off for either. No one is born good at skiing; some decide to continue to get better, while others do not.

Skål (sk-ull): a Norwegian word for 'cheers' or 'good health' – a salute or a toast, as to an admired person or group. They'll understand it if they're Danish, Swedish, Faroese or Icelandic.

So, take a deep breath, think about your job or your profession and ask yourself if you're getting caught up with someone else's metrics for success or if you are being true to your own. If I were to compare my hobby with those who are the best at it, within a hundredth of a second I could go from content to disheartened. Whose rules are you playing by? Whose blueprint are you following? Yours or someone else's?

Sunk Cost Fallacy Revisited

No matter how much you have already invested, only your assessment of the future costs and benefits counts.

Rolf Dobelli

For those who have not read *Not a Diet Book*, the sunk cost fallacy is where people struggle to walk away from something due to the amount of time, money or effort already invested in it. But these factors should not hold weight in any decision-making process around continuing or discontinuing whatever it is you're currently invested in, whether that be a person or a profession.

If you invested 10 per cent of your savings in stocks two years ago, but they haven't moved more than 1 per cent since then, do you feel obliged to hold on to them or to let them go? I bet in your head you'd be leaning towards keeping them – it's been two years of waiting for them to increase in value, so why waste that amount of time, right?

Or take a marriage. It is based on partnership, on love, on happiness and wanting to share the great moments of life together, yet so many are unhappy. Why? The kids? Well, although yes, I agree, separated parents can be more dysfunctional than those together, surely two happy adults apart would be more functional than two unhappy ones living together under one roof? So, why do so many stay together? Because they've already invested so much in the marriage. Therefore, the decision is made based on the time spent in the relationship or the marriage, not the quality of it.

I know I made this point in my first book, but it's important to make it clear again. You must only make judgements based on where you are at now, not where you were at previously and not where you might be. This is living in the present. The past no longer exists and it's time you came to terms with that reality. What has happened occurred when the rock we live on was in a different part of the universe, and it will never revisit that location. To believe otherwise is naive.

THE MONTY HALL PROBLEM

Here's a prime example of our fear around making decisions when the outcome is partly unknown: there are three doors, one of which has your favourite car behind it, while the other two have goats behind them. I let you pick any one of the three doors, and once you have selected it, I pick one of the other two (I know where the goats are). I open a door to show you a goat, and I then give you the opportunity to switch doors: do you take the switch? In most cases, you won't. People don't. They hold on tighter to their initial choice, even though more information is available to them. Your odds of winning go from 33 per cent to 66 per cent in what is known as 'the Monty Hall problem' if you switch. But although the odds are doubled in the case of switching, only around 13 per cent of people choose to do so given the opportunity. (See References, p. 255.)

Your future is malleable, but I don't want you to plan for that either. To be a future-planning person could cause you to neglect the present. **Your today constructs your tomorrow.** So, don't try to step ahead or jump past a crucial step which is right now. The future is not in your full control, your past has happened, so you're only left with right now. To make judgements based on your past is to make the same mistake as millions do each and every fucking day, falling victim to the sunk cost fallacy, remaining invested in the past and not the present. It sounds stupid to remind you but I think it's fitting that I do – to remind you that you cannot change your past, you can't fix what went wrong, you can't worry about the situation that happened and you can't let it affect you now; you can't wear your failures of the past in the present. Every day is a page in a book: you should never turn back a page, or skip a chapter or worry about what is on the page to come; just stay focused on the page in hand and enjoy each and every line for itself.

So, make decisions based on now, on today, on the second you read this. Do you love your partner right now? Do you want to remain with them longer right now? Do you love your job right now? Stop thinking about how long you have been there; whether a month or a tenure, you can only let today influence your decision, not the amount of time invested. Don't let the sunk cost fallacy take hold.

There are millions of people losing millions in currency, millions of unhappy marriages and unhappy relationships and millions of investments turning sour because people are too caught up in how long they've been invested in them. I know that divorce costs a fortune, but think of the cost of living an unhappy life or wasting time – the most valuable commodity of all.

Realize that sleeping on a futon* when you're thirty is not the worst thing. You know what's worse? Sleeping in a king bed next to a wife you're not really in love with but for some reason you married, and you got a couple kids, and you got a job you hate. You'll be laying there fantasizing about sleeping on a futon. There's no risk when you go after a dream. There's a tremendous amount to risk to playing it safe.

Bill Burr

Many people think of the solar system as being still, the sun chilling in the middle and the planets orbiting. But our solar system moves at around 828,000 km an hour around the Milky Way. It will take us about 230 million years to do a full orbit of that bad boy. So, guess what? That time you messed up really badly last week? We're now at least 139,104,000 km from that point; it only remains a part of your identity if you choose to let it. We're 240 million years away from even getting close to where that happened again in the next galaxy orbit, so don't treat it like it's in your DNA; it's a part of the past. The universe continually moves on, so I suggest you do, too.

There are hard decisions to make today that will inevitably get put off until tomorrow and this will be the downfall of millions of people today, and then again the next day, and the next, I'm sure. Are you going to be one of those people? Well, that's up to you, isn't it? Turn this page very carefully – because what you do after reading it influences the trajectory of your life.

* Futon: a padded unsprung mattress originating in Japan that can be rolled up or folded in two.

The whole future lies in uncertainty: live immediately.

Seneca

The Power of the Anomaly

It's human nature to conjure the anomaly when a harsh truth is presented to us. If I said, 'Long-distance relationships don't work,' you'd straight away think of the rare couple out of everyone you know who made it work. This is the way our minds work and, unfortunately, we unknowingly make irrational decisions devoid of proper logic or pragmatism because of it.

Why I hate the lottery

Buying a lottery ticket, to me, belongs to the mindset of leaving luck to govern the outcome of your financial position. Not only do I find it a poor value to 'wish for' in life, I think that each time you buy a ticket you demotivate yourself in the actual pursuit of what you want in the subconscious belief that you can win it instead.

I've yet to think of a successful gambler off the top of my head. Sure, there may be a few that slide into my mind, but that's just the confirmation bias at play: I will swarm my mind with the few people who have won lots of money without really knowing how much they've lost or sacrificed behind closed doors. It's not often that you hear about the people who have lost everything to gambling either. Truth be told, I don't gamble at all, except for a fun poker night. The thing is, I don't like the mindset that goes with it.

The gambling mindset is: I will put what I can here and I *might* see a return.

'Might' is at very best, too. There are so many places we can put our efforts where we *will* see a return. They may not be as glamorous as a casino with a free drink (put into your hand every ten minutes by the waitress trying to get you drunk, as the oxygen in the casino keeps you wide awake three hours beyond the time you promised yourself you'd go home). Everyone is living for that big win, but for most it will never happen. They'll run out of time, money or both.

The human mind is very quick to conjure up the anomaly in most scenarios. When I say the sea is safe you will think of the last shark attack; when I say planes are safe you will think about the last plane to crash; when I say long-distance relationships are not a good idea you'll tell me about how Steve and Sandra managed to make it work and it's been ten years. Our brains can't quantify the stories of where it didn't happen; it's a lot less glamorous and a lot less memorable.

The confirmation bias is a phenomenon whereby human beings in charge of making a decision have been shown to actively seek out and assign more weight to evidence that confirms their existing idea or belief and ignore or discredit evidence to the contrary. So, if you already believe the sea is full of hungry sharks or the skies are full of falling planes, you won't listen or credit anything I bring to the table, as your mind has already been made up.

My advice is to ignore the lottery.* If you want a way out or a better quality of life, you'll need to work for it. Want a good place to invest

---

* I know a lot of people become triggered about my anti-lottery standpoint. They say, 'But the charity does great things.' Well, if you're that much of a philanthropist, you could just donate direct to a charity on a regular basis without random people pocketing millions in the process.

£10? Try a book instead of a scratch-card. The lottery winners are paraded in the news to feed your bias, to summon up the anomaly in front of your eyes, to deceive you into thinking you stand a chance. Don't stand for it. Don't expect someone to come along and make it easy – because that goes against how the universe works.

The chances of winning the UK lottery jackpot are 1 in 45,057,474. (See References, p. 255.) From both a mindset and a statistical perspective, I'd say don't let a bit of paper, a collection of random numbers and chance have a hold on the direction of your ambition. If you want something to change, you're in the driver's seat of your life. So, pick the direction and put your foot down.

Basically, stop believing in the lottery and start believing in yourself.

But why is it that our minds work like this? They have been programmed to do so, that's why. Think about this for a second: why is it that when we buy a lottery ticket, we get butterflies in our stomachs believing we might win? But on the other hand, when we think about swimming in the sea we worry about sharks. How on earth can we make such irrational assumptions at different ends of a spectrum? Statistically speaking, the probability of either eventuality is very low, and yet we hedge our bets on one, while being afraid of the other. It's a paradoxical thought process that we're not questioning. Neither of these things is within our control at all. (Bar buying multiple tickets or swimming in colder waters, you cannot influence them.) It's like when turbulence rocks the plane you are on and the seatbelt light turns on, you think you're about to die and how tragic it is that your last meal was on a plane. I know because I've felt it, too.

And here's the really crazy thing: we put more trust and belief in things that are extremely unlikely to happen than in those we can actually control. If you want to earn more money, why not just ask for a pay rise? Why not charge more for your services or start a side hustle? If

I was to be a pessimist and say there was only a 5 per cent chance of your boss agreeing to such terms, you'd still be tens of thousands of times more likely to get the pay increase than you would be of winning the lottery. A small bump in your salary would probably involve less anxiety around where to spend your money or who your real friends are than lottery winners no doubt contend with. And charging more for your services means you can work fewer hours and earn more money. Yet we're petrified and scared of the failure that could result. Why do we overestimate the chances of a plane crash, shark attack or lottery win when there are things we can do right now that are thousands of times more likely to yield a positive outcome?

Exchange rates and balancing acts

There's a currency we can all use which means you don't need to worry about exchange rates as you travel overseas. That currency is one the richest can still be poor with. That currency is happiness.

Have you ever realized that happiness doesn't change in value as you cross borders, time zones or continents? Happiness is invisible and so we struggle to quantify it: we can't count it, we can't stack it up, we can't give it to those who need it and we can't win it by chance or save it up for when we may need it. Money, on the other hand, isn't influenced by who you're with, your perspective on a current situation or where your mental health is – yet we place so much importance on it.

Don't get me wrong. Money is important. But it's not the be all and end all.

We've all been there job hunting, salary-driven and hungry for a bigger payslip. We all daydream about what we could buy, where we could live and how it would feel to buy dinner for all of our loved ones.

Money is great. But we always need to think about the toll it takes on other areas of our lives that will impact our level of happiness.

Other factors we need to consider within the currencies of money and happiness include working hours, shift patterns, stress, work–life balance and environment. By no means do we want an easy ride; I mean, adversity is welcome and often to be cherished. I think J. Willard Marriott says it best when he says:

> *Good timber does not grow with ease; the stronger the wind, the stronger the trees.*
>
> J. Willard Marriott (founder of Marriott Hotels)

If we look at growing muscles, we need stress, we need damage and we need to give them the well-earned break they need to grow and develop – because there is always a turning point at which you can train too much and it has a diminishing return. Finding the sweet spot calls for the ability to dial up when you want to and to ease off when required. Some professions, and often the higher-paid jobs, do not take into account a good work–life balance. Have you ever considered whether you are getting a fair transaction in the work–life balance? Are you giving a huge part of your life away for marginal returns in terms of freedom, happiness and wellbeing? Or perhaps you're actually giving too little for your monetary return because you're not happy where you are? Wherever you are on this spectrum, I want you to think about whether you consider this balance to be meaningful to you. The sweet spot requires freedom and it requires you, in some circumstances, to look beyond just the salary – like a fitness person seeking the optimal environment for muscle growth, you must do the same with your work.

It takes effort to reject the status quo and detach ourselves from the norm, no longer following the herd and seeing the highest salary as the epitome of working life. But if we become environment-driven rather than salary-driven, **if we seek a multi-currency approach, including satisfaction and both financial and environmental fulfil- ment, we can create and build a life that serves growth** rather than a purely financial figure. Someone with a great work–life balance on an average salary is far wealthier than a stressed, tired and overworked millionaire. Always keep that in mind.

Individual Values

I get asked most days why I became a personal trainer in the first place. Truth be told, my sister texted me one day saying, 'Why don't you become a PT?' I was hell-bent on regaining my fitness after travelling in Southeast Asia, knowing how much it was going to hurt getting back to the first game of rugby. I became the chicken-and-broccoli-wielding wanker, doing my best to get a grip back on my life, and my sister noted before I did that I could make a living from it.

I thought to myself: me? A personal trainer? Firstly, of course, my mind flooded with self-doubt: I'd inevitably be a failure; I'd not stuck with any job for more than a year; my dating history was just as dire. But as I thought about it, one thing was apparent – that I'd no doubt enjoy it. Surely that would beat wearing a suit and sneaking off to the stationery cupboard, grabbing a handful of Mentos from the bowl that resided in one of the dreary offices on the way.

I thought long and hard and came to realize a few things: I could wear shorts to work, talk to people all day, get a good step count in and, in the event that I got enough clients, it would be a dreamy job, perhaps something for the interim until I figured out which direction I really wanted to go in life. Little did I know that within four years all of what I thought was possible was about to change. I would be considered one of the most successful personal trainers ever to come out of the United Kingdom, or even Australia, for that matter.

I remember living off near to nothing in Asia; I was happy, carefree and stress-free, although I admit, it is hard to have a work–life balance without work. I came to see that I could work a handful of hours, pay my car finance and afford nights out with my rugby team (I always joked that my drinking team had a big rugby problem). There were days when my alarm went off at 5 a.m. and, before I knew it, I had this crazy sensation as I arrived at the front door of the gym that I'd never felt before: I actually enjoyed my work.

I think self-development is at the heart of taking the initial plunge and making the associated effort to improve in your line of work, then reaping the satisfaction that comes with it. To me, I never truly wanted to be a good recruiter or a good IT sales rep, as I didn't enjoy my work; I didn't want to get better at something I didn't want to do. I think when people hit a brick wall in their profession and they're not sure where to go it's because on a subconscious level they may not want to do it any more. But they then fall victim to the sunk cost fallacy.

We're made to feel like we can't control our values, but we honestly can. Twin boys can grow up, same birth date, same address, same height, same weight, play the same sport and even enjoy the same video games. However, as they grow older, it will become apparent what those boys value and cherish, whether that's recognition, praise, accomplishments, how they dress or how they're perceived by others. Values are really unique to who we are and what we deem important, and it's often hard to know what they are until we're really questioned on them.

So right now, I ask you: what is important to you? Think about it. Because if you put down this book to check your Instagram feed, chances are you value that higher than this book. I bet some of the values that come to mind would be the normal 'being kind to people', 'being generous', 'being a good citizen' … But do your actions back that up? What do you do on a daily basis that would be good evidence of that? Probably not as much as you think, I'd bet.

We are walking, talking manifestations of our values. The way we interact, react – all of it is based around the values we are currently striving for. It's interesting because when I mentioned my little midlife crisis, people jokingly said I was 'finding myself'; but really I was re-aligning myself with new and fresh values. The eyes through which I saw the world were different and then, and only then did I realize what was important to me and, ultimately, what wasn't.

I can't help but think that so many people have slotted into their current values by default, often via parents and the education system, and no one is telling them any different. You can love your parents and what they stand for – I do, wholeheartedly – but I cannot share their values. The world is a different place now from what it was a generation ago. Think of it this way: our parents, despite how much they love and care for us, quite literally lived a different life from ours today. The way we live is changing much faster than the values we can potentially inherit. This isn't to say that you shouldn't listen to your parents – but be careful to choose your own values. Otherwise, it could be like trying to put a cassette tape into a CD player.

We must not live our lives pursuing the values of the rest of the herd, because there's every chance that a large proportion of that herd are living a life of quiet misery and desperation in the mistaken belief that they're broken, when actually it's just that the blueprint isn't suited to them.

Controlling values: the subjective nature of good vs bad

Subjective is an adjective and it means 'based on or influenced by personal feelings, tastes or opinions'. It sits on the opposite end of the spectrum to objective, which represents hard facts. Here's another way to think about it: imagine if we burned every book and study that existed so nothing remained. In time, I'm sure gravity would be 'discovered' with the same outcome, as would particle physics and the speed of sound and light, all with the same conclusions as before. However, if all documentation of religion, for example, were to be removed, I imagine it would all come back a little differently. Objectively speaking, 100 degrees Celsius is the boiling point of water at sea level. That's not influenced by how you feel about it; that's what science tells us, and being science-minded is to seek the objective truth. On the other hand, if I was to say that Eric Prydz was one of the best DJs ever, that's not objectively speaking. It's just my opinion, therefore subjective (my parents would probably disagree strongly and say, 'It's just noise').

Now, going off on a tangent slightly, something I learned recently is that the higher you take water, the lower its boiling point. If you go to the top of Mount Everest, water will boil at 71 degrees Celsius. (The higher you go, the less the atmospheric pressure, therefore the lower the boiling point.) Titan, one of Saturn's largest moons, is one of the only other places in our solar system with liquid on its surface besides Earth. However, the seas there are made up of ethane and methane, which are both gases on Earth.

The reason I bring this up is because things can be vastly different in different places but also be the same. For instance, values in one place might be positive, yet the same thing elsewhere may not be. It's individual and ultimately subjective to each person. In the UK, staying late at work may show your new boss that you're a hard worker, but in another country and culture (like Germany), it could imply that you're not using your time productively enough.

Whether something is good or bad for someone is based upon their individual circumstances – there are no one-size-fits-all values, although we've seen them idealized in various religions over the years. I can only imagine that the Ten Commandments were an incredibly smart idea for instilling values in people at the time with a pinch of scare tactics: abide by these values or a man in the sky will not be happy; you can't see him but he created all this, so don't piss him off by stealing from your neighbour, all right?

Is running good? Well, for a young athlete, of course. For my ninety-seven-year old nan, no it's not. Is coffee good? Well, at 6 a.m., yes. At 9 p.m., no, as it will more than likely disrupt your sleep. Similarly, when we are thinking about values, ultimately, we want them to align with what is right for us, right now, and with how the repercussions of holding them will serve us over time.

A very important aspect of the values we hold is the extent to which we can control them. In my early years, I was very money-focused, and I held dear what I earned and what my future earnings could be. Now, money is a pretty poor value, but worst of all, it's very difficult to control. The COVID-19 pandemic sent a shockwave through the world's economy – in a matter of weeks, stocks were gone and employment down, as businesses had to close.

If you allow money to be the sole source of what brings you happiness, you are leaving your fate in someone else's hands. Money is an uncontrollable variable which could, depending on circumstances (such as a recession or a global pandemic), leave you feeling like you have nothing to be happy for and therefore nothing to live for. It sounds pretty fucked, but **if you have a value you can't control, it could all too easily end up controlling you**.

One really important value for me on a personal level is my freedom each day to have time to myself. Funnily enough, when things go great for me, I feel my freedom impaired. Whether it's TV appearances, radio shows or PR discussions, suddenly my calendar fills up and there's very little I can do to change it. Then I feel slightly suffocated, even though I do appreciate their importance. On the other hand, when things are quiet and I'm forced into self-isolation and social distancing,* I sit back and experience a wealth of happiness, as I am completely free to do whatever I want. Whether that's masturbation, a random shower to come up with a good idea or a stint on a gaming console, I value my freedom highly.

Many people who seek freedom think an impressive financial status automatically provides it. But I don't think it does. It all too often means more worries, more leeches wanting a piece of your pie and, ultimately, more taxes to pay on nearly everything you can imagine.

In ethics, values are a sign of the degree of importance we attach to a thing or an action. This helps us decide what to do and how we want to live. **Don't think about *what you want* in life; instead put some thought into *how you want to live*** – what you cherish and what you feel is important – and align that with what makes you, the individual, happy. Every person on the planet is different; we may all belong to the same species, but even identical twins have different needs and wants for their time on Earth.

---

* As I very much doubt that COVID-19 is going to be the only viral disease of our time, I think we should shift the emphasis of the terminology to 'physical distancing' rather than 'social distancing', as the last thing we want is to distance socially; we're all human and incredibly social by nature.

> **TASK**
>
> Write down ten values you hold dear and examine them. Then look at your day-to-day actions and determine whether or not these align with your values, and whether you need a change in values or a change in lifestyle. Identify uncontrollable values and perhaps those you hold dear because of the influence of other people.

I followed my own fitness journey, and that led me on to the path of becoming a personal trainer thanks to my sister's advice. But all roads must lead to job satisfaction; even if you're not passionate about the business per se, there must be an element of happiness. For example, you may not be passionate about selling swimming-pool filters, but if your business allows you to get out of bed at 10 a.m., work for four hours, then go walk your dogs on the beach, you might well be very happy and therefore passionate about your work because of the structure it has given you.

It's not a figure, a sum, a mortgage or a credit rating. It's not the 0–60 mph of your car or the brand of watch you're wearing. It's not where you sit on a plane or the hotel you stay in. Happiness in your work life is a strange sensation and nothing conveys it better than this:

Happiness is wanting what you already have.

Lucy Lord, great friend and even better baker

When the components of your existing working life contribute to whatever you could ever want from a work–life balance, then – and only then – can you sit back and experience the same feeling I have had in my time as a personal trainer. You can have all the money in the world, but if you don't have satisfaction from your work it'd be like turning up to Wimbledon's centre court without a racquet or any balls.

Time

We're unsure if time is finite or infinite. For a start, it's also relative, so we could get very lost in philosophical debate on the universe or whether the Big Bang, as we know it, was the first of its kind or one of many. However, one thing is for sure: **our time on the planet is finite**. The amount of time we exist on the revolving ball of mass known as planet Earth is governed by where we are born, what our parents do, how they set our thinking and values, how we perceive them, how we live our lives, what we prioritize and, of course, a big dose of sheer fucking luck. Because you could have everything going for you as far as being set up to do well is concerned, but all it takes is to be in the wrong place at the wrong time and that finite amount of time is up.

Einstein's theory of relativity still blows my mind, but even if I briefly explain what relativity is, imagine this: you and I are on a train and the train is travelling at 100 mph. We're standing at either end of the carriage; I then throw a ball to you at 10 mph. To us, on the train, the ball is moving at just 10 mph, but to someone on the platform as the train goes by, they observe the ball moving at 110 mph. However, there is no such thing as absolute rest for anyone in the scenario, as the planet is constantly rotating in orbit around the sun. Therefore, 'time' is relative to the person experiencing it.

I could get into the physics of how time slows for anything approaching the speed of light. However, I'm not here to try to knock Stephen Hawking off the top spot in the astrophysics book charts any time soon. The point I want to make clear is that we must approach life understanding that the time we have (relative or not) and the life we live are finite.

· But before looking at the time we have on the planet, let's first have a round of applause for how lucky you are. Not just that you found my book, but because you're alive in the first place. I remember at school saying to some of my classmates, 'A hundred-thousand sperm and *you* were the fastest?' But not just that. Rewind further still: life itself. We are so lucky to have evolved from a single-cell organism to a bunch of organized apes.

When I talk about time across space, I know you'll probably be thinking: aliens, other species out there. But here it is: our solar system is unique compared to many others. Planet Earth was left alone for around three billion years, allowing single-cell organisms to become life. That's a quarter of the time since the Big Bang – a lot of time when you think of it. Not only that, if the asteroid that caused the dinosaurs to become extinct hadn't come, we could be right now hiding from a Tyrannosaurus rex. I'm not going to lie to you, I love going off on tangents when I write, so here's my final one for this chapter: dinosaurs, right? We have their fossils to know their sizes. For instance, we know that the Tyrannosaurus rex was up to 20 feet tall, but how do we know what sounds they make? How did they come up with that for *Jurassic Park*? I'll leave you to think about that one.

So, we're pretty unique to have evolved into life. Although there is almost definitely life in other areas of the cosmos, I think we're one of the very few life forms with the ability **to think about our existence** and other life surrounding us. On a separate note, for any of you paranoid that aliens are watching us, they'd have to be within a spherical distance of less than 150 light years to see any of our advancements since we invented electricity. Which is very close. If there was life near the centre of our own Milky Way, they'd be over 25,000 light years away. This means that if they were eyeing up humans on planet Earth from where they are in relation to us, they'd see us hunting woolly mammoths.

So, not only are we hugely fortunate from a space and a sperm perspective, we're also hugely fortunate from a lifestyle perspective. Whether you're reading this in hardback, ebook or audiobook format, you're luckier than most other humans on Earth. To be able to read, let alone have a smart device, puts you ahead of everyone else who doesn't have that ability. I'm grateful you're reading this, too. Remember, **those who *don't* read have no advantage over those who *can't* read.** I like to remind people of this when they shun the idea of a good book. When we look at how fortunate we are in our lives, it's apparent that luck plays a huge part of it. For instance, the month you're born can have a huge part to play in whether or not you make it as an athlete; in the same school year there can be 364 days' age difference between two pupils, and the development that can occur in that time can mean everything for them when playing the same position in their sport. It could mean the difference between being selected for an academy or not. Malcom Gladwell makes this very clear in the book *Outliers*: those who go to the academies will almost definitely be on a faster trajectory to the 10,000 hours of mastery.*

> *It is those who are successful, in other words,*
> *who are most likely to be given the kinds of special*
> *opportunities that lead to further success.*
>
> Malcolm Gladwell, in *Outliers: The Story of Success*

---

* Gladwell (in *Outliers*) explains the 10,000-hour Rule, which he considers the key to success in any field; it is simply a matter of practising a specific task that can be accomplished, for instance, with twenty hours of work a week for ten years.

The point I want to make clear is this: to even be worrying and having this discussion about our time is a miracle in itself. It's a finite blink of existence across something so much bigger than us and it's not to be taken for granted, ever. I'm not your time-management guru; I don't come armed with PDFs showing how to make your time 'work for you'. But I am here to tell you that time is getting away from you … well, all the time. Whenever I had a group of friends at university who didn't want to go out, I'd always say to them, 'Today is the oldest you've ever been and also the youngest you'll ever be!' It's a good way to get people to do something they may not want to do (such as join you for two-for-one cocktails on a school night).

Hence my angst when someone spends their time doing something they don't enjoy. Everyone loves to think we're some form of divine inter-vention, but we're not – we're a long line of miracles over time. Billions of years of colliding rocks, incredible statistical chances and anomalies did not merge over such a long time span for you to wake up each day not enjoying the time you were blessed with in the first place. Usually the best-paid jobs consume us the most and we're trading **our time + our lives** for money. It's essential you get a good deal – one that can't be measured in finance, but can only be quantified in terms of your enjoy-ment of the finite time you're given. The paradox is that finite thinking within a finite timeframe can be hard to combat in the moment: when we're hot, we forget what it is like to be cold. When we're cold, we forget what it's like to be hot. When we're angry, we forget what it's like to be calm, and when we're calm, we forget what it's like to be angry.

This is, of course, why I think meditation has such profound effects on people's mental wellbeing. It is a daily practice whereby people set aside time for themselves, for nothing, for clarity, for thoughts without distraction; sitting down and giving themselves the gift that not many people choose to: time itself.

Meditation

I have a section on my phone labelled 'advice not to fall on deaf ears'. In that section, I write down advice I'm given, and considering how selective I am with who I spend time with, it's more often than not quite simply great advice. I take it, even if it's a bit late, and when I do, I generally end up pestering my friends to follow suit, hoping my advice doesn't fall on deaf ears.

> **TASK**
>
> Create a notes section on your phone. Call it 'advice not to fall on deaf ears'. Now, whether you follow it or not, at least write it down. One day you'll think about what to watch, buy or learn from and you can just go to that list.

Now, I'm going to write this entire section of the book without using the 'M' word, because to me it's an instant NOPE from my brain. I can imagine some dude in leggings telling me I need to get my 'medi on bro' and that my Warrior II is far too stiff. I'm well aware that most of the best minds in the world do it. But sometimes you have to make something sexy for people to do it. Let me explain.

So, we know that the key to fat loss is to 'eat less and move more', but we need to spice things up occasionally and make them sexy for the person who needs to do them. That's why we see so much love for trends like 'intermittent fasting'. It's no longer a case of just eating less and moving more. That's far too reductive, too common, too bland. Now it's fasting, it's intermittent and it's revolutionary – it's going to help you live longer, it's going to cure you of any disease. Well, that's bullshit, but you see where I am going. And I know from experience that if I told you to do the 'M' word, you probably wouldn't, but if I could make it sexy, you just might.

You're busy, too busy, your mind is too active, you may have kids or a busy job, or even better yet, you *don't have time* … But what if I told you that all I wanted from you was to spend ten minutes a day doing nothing? That's it. It can be when you wake up, when the sun is out and you sit on the doorstep outside your house; it can be when you wait for your kids in the car outside school. It could be anywhere. Just ten minutes. In those ten minutes you think about your tasks for the day, your priorities, your state of mental health, what's been making you unhappy, what's been making you happy, maybe you need to come up with an idea for something and be creative.

Surely being creative benefits your day? Now, suddenly, you're beginning to realize that's exactly what you need – as you're thinking through all of these important topics you empty your mind, listen to your breath and just let your mind wander. This is when I get the major-ity of my best ideas. I do it sometimes sitting, sometimes walking and very often in the shower. I just enjoy the feeling of the shower and take ten minutes in there (to the annoyance of my flatmates who need to get ready for work) as I become a silent (and well washed) philosopher.

With our time, I think it's important that we occasionally apply a change in perspective to its already finite nature. What if you had a week, a year or five years left? Would you do things differently? Why is that?

> **TASK**
>
> Grab your phone and use Siri (or Google Assistant) and say, 'Remind me tomorrow to "take ten",' then select a time and put ten minutes aside. This is not negotiable. Enjoy and thank me later for what you get from it.

Whatever you want to do, do it now. There are only so many tomorrows.

Michael Landon

Vivre pour toujours …

… meaning 'to live for ever' in French. Why French? Because it looks clichéd as hell in English!

I know it's a morbid subject, but that's the point. Some think we're not far off the technology to live for ever. I think that's about as daft as holding out for a lottery ticket. They say nothing is certain in life apart from death and taxes, and I think they're right. I think we need to talk about death more often because it's important to be pragmatic about it. You will die, just as surely as that your next holiday will come to an end. That's not to say you should worry about how long you're on holiday for, just how to treat each day. And instead of fearing *growing* old, we should be very grateful for *being* old, as it means we haven't died yet. I talk later in this book about the notion of seeing a sunset somewhere in the world on holiday and that you may not see that sunset there again, and that in itself is what makes the fabric of life so unique and so brilliant.

You ever noticed that when a tree dies it doesn't complain, it just makes way for another one, and the tree's decay is what gives nourishment to the next.

There are two questions I hate that I'm often asked about death: the first is, 'James, what would your death-row meal be?' Now, firstly, I hope not to be on death row. I don't plan on going to jail, thank you very much. Also, why the hell should the fact that I'm dying change what I want to eat for dinner? I don't think the news that I was about to get the lethal injection would increase my appetite for a particular cuisine. Not only that, but if you're getting the death penalty, why on earth do you get the choice of what to have for dinner? My dad wasn't even given that right by my mum! The second question is about knowing you only have a certain amount of time to live. For instance, 'If you had a week to live, what would you do?' People at this moment leak things they would want to do before they die. Now, here's the issue in my eyes: that these things aren't being planned for in any case, right now.

Let's say someone says, 'I'd do a dream trip to Hawaii and surf.' Then why aren't they planning for that now? Why does it have to take impending death for them to do it? What if someone said swimming with dolphins or to see the Great Wall of China? Why is their ultimate pursuit kept in a dream state, only to be unlocked by the prospect of death? Why not keep that idea in your thoughts now, *in the present*? I mean, it's only a morbid thought if you choose to see it that way. In the right context, it could be motivating, almost a trigger for Parkinson's law.*

As an example, take the idea of cleaning the house: when you have twenty minutes to clean, a lot gets done vs the time you had all day

---

* Parkisnon's law is the adage that 'work expands so as to fill the time available for its completion'.

and nothing got cleaned. It's a bit like the training session that took an hour and you spent the majority of it scrolling on social media, as opposed to when you had twenty minutes in the gym and couldn't walk for days afterwards. I think it can be appropriate to draw this adage into life: it will end, there is a finite capacity for life to be lived, and even if we did have the technological advancements for extended life, it wouldn't save you from a bus when you crossed the road too hastily without doing your due diligence for oncoming traffic.

Over the years, people have found so many different ways to be at peace with the concept of death, the end of life, whether through religion or stoicism, etc. Many of them have deemed it the beginning of life, and while I'm not so sure that's a safe bet to put all your chips on, I do often wonder who is at more peace – those who see it coming or those who don't? Humans by nature hugely underestimate bad things happening to them. Please don't skim over that last sentence. One more time: *hugely underestimate.* I'm not here to depress you, but those people who get a diagnosis of cancer, a rare brain tumour or end up in a near-fatal car crash woke up that day expecting everything to go right, to go to plan, to end the same as every other day before. This isn't to instil anxiety in you. It's to start an internal monologue of what if next week, next month, next year you got the news – would you be ready? For many people, there's this naivety that even if they did get the news, they'd have a year or six months to splurge their savings and enough energy to fulfil their bucket list. I think that naivety could be their downfall. I've never had a real written-down bucket list, but I have already easily done ten of fifteen things I'd love to do in life and the more of them that I've accomplished, the more at peace I can feel, not just with death, but life, too. It's not a hippie or spiritual thing, either; it's simply that if the news came that I didn't have as long as I thought I did, that would be OK.

Stemming from my values, which are very much driven by wanting to make the people around me proud, I feel fulfilled at my stage in life. But it hasn't always been this way. Rewind a handful of years and I would have said something very different. In as little as 10 per cent of my life I have managed to find this peace, this idea of being OK with the 'bad news'. Given the opportunity, would you rather spend your time between now and getting that news going for it, struggling, waking up at 5 a.m. and throwing everything you have to give at something, or just doing what everyone else does?

Whether it's launching a business, starting a martial art, a podcast or even a blog, there is no failure in going after a passion. The only way you can even feel you're not doing well is to either compare to someone else (comparison being the thief of joy) or to use someone else's values for measuring success. You may not get a blue tick (someone else's value), you may not get invited on to *The Ellen DeGeneres Show* (someone else's value). You may not even be able to fully support yourself financially with this passion, but that's not to say you won't in time. Although the only things for certain in life are death and taxes, you cannot afford to use that as the rule you live your life by.

> *If you want to live a happy life, tie it to a goal,*
> *not to people or things.*
>
> Albert Einstein

PART III
FOUNDATIONS

I know it sounds like a cliché that so many people use simply having 'the right mindset' as the key to success, but quite frankly, I think the topic needs to be more of a wake-up call for people to really understand that they're not limited. You can graduate from university at twenty-one – either you get good grades or you don't – and in most cases that's you done. But I would like everyone to re-imagine learning, and see it not as something that's done from childhood to age twenty-one, but instead as early education being assisted and anything beyond it being unassisted – by which I mean you have to do it yourself.

The reason I say this is because it's not always the smartest at school who end up the smartest in life; it's often not the ones with the best grades who end up the most successful in life either. We often risk perceiving our mindset as being similar to the size of an engine in a car – a finite capacity for acceleration that cannot be stretched.

Mindset

We think we're limited when it comes to confidence, audacity and what we can accomplish. We seem to think that we're stuck with that for the entirety of our lives, as though our potential is somehow pre-determined, and therefore it's more about dealing with that than about developing ourselves into a better and more successful version of ourselves. For some reason, we see ourselves in a mould – a bit like putty – and the mould solidifies in our younger years, so that by the time university finishes it's set, and it can't be shaped or changed. This idea is wrong. The notion of not being able to 'teach an old dog new tricks' has been dispelled; it's bullshit. It's imperative that you appreciate the malleability of your identity, intelligence and persona – they only set and harden if you believe that they will.

For example, the American music critic Harold Schonberg said that Mozart 'developed late' and that he didn't produce his greatest work until he'd had over twenty years of composing experience.

Education

It's also safe to say that we haven't cracked the education system yet. Finland, for instance, has one of the world's best education systems, whereby students not only enter it older than anywhere else, as late as the age of seven, they also have shorter learning days than most other countries.

Finland's education system works because its entire structure has been built around several core principles. First and foremost, equal access to education is a constitutional right. Another important principle is that one should be allowed to choose their educative path, which should never lead to a dead end.*

The part of this that's so important to me is that they allow students to choose their 'educative path'. Many of us are not given the same privilege and, ultimately, we can be led down a path to a dead end in education, which means we think it's time to stop learning. Once we stop learning, we feel like the mould of our intellectual identity begins to solidify and before you know it, we've hopped on that blueprint for life, travelling the trajectory of our 'qualifications', whether GCSEs, A levels or a degree.

What pains me the most is the thought that the subjects I was learning as a very young child didn't interest me, therefore I was classified as having 'learning difficulties', and from then on, I was automatically put in the bottom tier of education, even for work that was very easy for me. I was never stretched, challenged or given the choice to do or accomplish more. Once labelled with the inability to learn well, I was very much moulded into my 'set' at school and that's where I remained.

When I went to school, unfortunately a part of my brain began to die. I'm not sure if it was the part that became interested in girls, but I felt then that I wasn't right for school or education; I now realize that school and education weren't right for me. The entire system didn't work for me and nothing stimulated me to want to learn any of the subjects. It was only later, in my twenties, that I found that things began to align. I began to read more and instead of a thirst to play video

* See References, p. 255.

games, I developed a thirst for learning. I suddenly understood, ten years after leaving school, that I did, in fact, enjoy learning. I have since come to see that everyone loves learning; it just has to be the right things for the person. There are so many excellent fucking books to read. Why on earth *Of Mice and Men* made the school curriculum is beyond my understanding. It's quite literally the worst book I've read to date.

Being open to learning something each and every day has not only influenced what I learn and how I learn it, but, as a by-product, my wealth (not income) and my quality of life (and that of my friends and family) have also greatly improved. All because I developed a love for learning that influenced my perception, actions, ethos and ability to do certain things each day, which, as I soon found out, transformed who I was then into who I am now. And the best bit is, every ounce of knowledge was entirely self-taught. I am just someone of normal intelligence who enjoys the feeling of that eyebrow raise when you read something interesting. That's it, that's all I chase. That moment when you drop your shoulders and think: wow, isn't that interesting? If I get at least one of those a day, it makes me happy.

I have become hugely fascinated by learning and failing, two occurrences so often seen as being at different ends of the spectrum: one is being able to do something through the process of learning it, while the other is where we assume we can't be successful and that any pursuit of it will end in failure. Again, we are led to believe that we are not able to continue with learning and that brain development stops when we leave school. Part of this mindset is to do with the education system, and learning often being treated as a hurdle to get over, an exam to pass and a box to tick, and as a result of this, I believe that many people begin to see it almost as a punishment. School is the opposite of a holiday, so therefore learning is seen as the opposite of fun and freedom. The irony of this is that learning is the ultimate tool in giving us our freedom and leading us on to the path to fulfilment.

I can remember leaving school and I thinking at the time that the period of learning in my life was now over. I look back now and realize how wrong that was. Human beings are inquisitive and from a young age, I remember always wanting to know how something worked. I was always pulling my toys apart and wanting to know how they functioned. If you tell a child not to go somewhere, you'll inevitably find them there later; they go from not wanting to know to *needing to know.**

Sleep and brain function

During adolescence, especially puberty, we change not only physically through spurts of very fast growth and development, but in our brains, too. When my dad first noticed my voice had dropped, I said, 'No, it hasn't. I just have a cold.' Three weeks later, he said, 'How's your cold?' and I realized he was, in fact, right – in the space of a few days I had developed a completely different voice. Brain changes in adolescence are a big topic for discussion right now. If you're ever going to do something stupid, the likelihood is it will be in your teenage years. Neuroscientific debates are ongoing about when we should let

---

* My knowledge of nutrition and training – almost the entirety of *Not a Diet Book* – came from my wanting to learn the functions of the human body, anatomy and biomechanics. It wasn't that I wanted to learn all of it, but I needed to so I could be satisfied – just like when I was a child pulling apart those toys, I was now an adult delving into study through podcasts, books and audiobooks. I think that's simply human nature, but I feel that perhaps not enough people realize it.

teenagers drive or what the right age is to serve in the military. With the vast changes that take place in brain function and structure, we not only need perhaps a different approach, with more empathy, but a better understanding of how teenagers function.

In my first book, I went into great detail about circadian rhythm and how feeding and sleeping sit within a daily cycle in our lives. Changes in time zones (jet lag) disrupt this rhythm and make us feel pretty rubbish. Teenagers not only have huge changes in mood and physiology, but also in their sleep cycles. On the one hand, they want to set their own bedtimes, usually to the annoyance of their parents who are yelling 'Go to bed'; then, on the flip side, they need to be woken up by their parents or they'd 'sleep the day away'. I feel if society could, in the future, adjust school timings to allow for this, while it might be incredibly strange to have certain years arriving later, it could have a profound effect on children's ability to learn, remember, behave and perform in their academic studies and their sports. Environments are so important for work; office set-ups are at the forefront of innovation, yet school systems, where future generations are bred, are exposed to a structure that can be detrimental to learning.

SLEEP CYCLES RECAP*

So, now I'm going to talk about something that all of us have – even our pets. It's a circadian rhythm – our bodies' cycle that allows us to fall asleep when we're tired, and prompts us to wake up in the morning. There are two hormones you need to know about here: cortisol and melatonin.

Cortisol

Cortisol is one of the hormones we produce to help us get out of bed; this is known as the 'cortisol awakening response'. Unfortunately, this is why, often, when you wake up hungover, or try to have a lie in at the weekend, you can't simply fall back to sleep when you want to. The rhythm plays to your advantage to get you out of bed and into work each day and you can't simply shut it off as easily as you can your alarm. Incidentally, you'll note on days you go to bed on time and don't set an alarm you'll wake up at roughly the same time. This is due to your sleep rhythm. We usually only oversleep an alarm if we've had a late night or have messed up our sleep rhythm through international travel. Throughout the day, cortisol maintains blood glucose (aka blood-sugar levels). In addition to its vital role in normal daily function, it is a key player in the stress response. In the presence of a physical or psychological threat, cortisol levels surge to provide the energy (and substrates) necessary to cope with stress-provoking stimuli or to escape from danger – otherwise known as the 'fight-or-flight'

---

* This is an excerpt from a section of *Not A Diet Book*, and I strongly recommend you read it to fully understand the importance and impact of a healthy sleep cycle for physical and mental wellbeing.

response. Unfortunately, in the modern world it is quite common for this hormone to do its job more than it should. Social media, worrying about emails, things popping off in the group chat on WhatsApp, even when you come home to watch a gripping TV series – these all play into your hormonal response from cortisol which can make it difficult to fall asleep.

Melatonin (mela-toe-nin)

Melatonin is the hormone that helps us fall asleep. Remember the first time you were told that caffeine would improve sports performance of any kind and it became your go-to every time you needed to perform well? Melatonin is the complete opposite and is your go-to when trying to sleep. Unfortunately, there are not so many external aids to help us fall asleep without having to look to sedation through things like alcohol – and even then, there's no guarantee you won't wake up halfway through that sleep due to your body and circadian rhythm thinking it's just a nap. Disturbed circadian rhythms are associated with sleep disorders and impaired health. So, what does melatonin do? Melatonin regulates circadian rhythms such as the sleep-wake rhythm and neuroendocrine rhythms. Ingestion of melatonin induces fatigue, sleepiness and a diminution of sleep latency. When circadian rhythms are restored, behaviour, mood, development, intellectual function, health and sometimes seizure control can improve. (See References, p. 255.)

When I was at school, I wanted to get the train with my dad in the mornings. I felt it was a lot 'cooler' and trendy to do so. It was about the feeling of being independent, and because my dad had to commute to work it meant getting up pretty early. The train was at 7 a.m., I didn't need to be at school until 9 a.m. and it was only a twenty-minute train ride. Looking back now, I was lucky to get five or six hours of sleep during secondary school and I do wonder if that was a big contributing factor to poor concentration and behaviour. I saw an educational psychologist, but not once did anyone wonder if I was simply not sleeping enough. A recent poll by the National Sleep Foundation found that over 45 per cent of adolescents in the United States obtain inadequate sleep due to a lack of societal empathy for changes that occur during development. (See References, p. 255)

As adults, we are all too aware that when we're tired, we feel like crap and we know we need to rest or do less. I think that when teenagers complain about sadness, fatigue or malaise, we should take into consideration their circadian rhythm changes that are only going to be further disrupted by the technology we have in the modern world, whether smartphones, televisions or gaming consoles.

In the 1990s, a study was performed in the United States about bedtimes set by parents:

The analysis showed that young people whose parent set their bedtime at midnight or after relative to those with bedtimes set at 22:00 or earlier, were significantly more likely to suffer from depression or suicidal ideation. The authors also found that this association was mediated by total sleep time; thus, those with earlier bedtimes reported sleeping more and were less likely to be depressed or experience suicidal ideation.*

* See References, p. 255.

There are other studies which conclude that a parental set bedtime will mean more sleep and therefore less daytime fatigue. Something as simple as having a fixed bedtime could have a profound impact on improving mental health, performance and the ability to learn and develop.

For anyone reading this book now, I have a feeling it may be a little bit late to get on to your parents about setting your bedtime. However, you're being armed with the knowledge about setting a bedtime. There are so many things that we're not able to control in life, but sleep is one that we can. I can't think of a time I've ever got someone to prioritize their sleep and they've regretted it. So, rather than blindly following society's expectations of what a good night's sleep is, you must take control and appreciate the return you could get from an investment as small as turning the TV off or putting your phone down that bit earlier (for you and also for those around you).

This is not a new-era way of thinking. These things have been studied for decades and it makes me wonder why we have not adapted to what we've suspected and known for so long. We can't expect society to do it for us. This again is another reason why, as a parent or even a future parent, you must get on top of the controllable variables at play here. Just because we've known something doesn't mean it's going to be changed anytime soon. Shift work is essential, we can't just switch off the world at night, and I have the utmost respect and gratitude for health workers and service workers all the way to highway-maintenance workers who sacrifice their sleep patterns for society to function. A slightly shifted school day for adolescents could not only reduce disruptions, poor behaviour and people 'bunking' classes, but it could have hugely beneficial positives on the other side. Imagine if you would that secondary school could start at 10:30 (ninety minutes later) and finish ninety minutes later. You could not only play into the physiology and development of young adults and future generations, but simultaneously let teachers have a little longer in bed each morning, not having to worry about the school 'rush-hour' traffic. There is such rigid adherence in society to the way things have been with not much look to the future; innovation is defined as 'to make changes in something established, especially by introducing new methods, ideas, or products'. Within education especially, I feel we still overlook innovation, which means that hundreds if not thousands of school attendees will feel how I did.

Limiting Beliefs

One of the biggest hurdles we face when thinking about the state of our current mindset is limiting beliefs and boundaries. We think that our capacity for growth, for intelligence and for success is finite and that things are set and governed by boundaries, which they are not; we then have a set of beliefs that back up and fortify our boundaries – what we can do, what we can't, what we're capable of doing and what we're not capable of doing.

Boundaries never physically exist unless we build them; even the boundaries between countries, states, counties and cities are made up and do not physically exist, so the ones in your mind are even less real.

What are limiting beliefs? To me they're constraints we impose on ourselves – both consciously and subconsciously. Something as simple as believing or assuming something that results in limited potential can have a huge and profound impact on what we do, what we say, how we act and, ultimately, what we achieve. There is no one source from which they derive. Many factors (including upbringing, parents, culture, education, experience or societal influence) combine to create our beliefs and understanding of the world and, most importantly, our place within it, and we then apply a faulty logic based on these to the scenarios we face in everyday life.

Whether we like to admit it or not, **fear is the underlying principle of limiting beliefs**. I will talk about fear in more depth in the next chapter; we fear what we don't understand, we fear failure, but we also fear success.

The Effort Paradox

One of my first limiting beliefs was about how much I could charge as a personal trainer on the gym floor. I set my pricing based on what other personal trainers were charging (classic herd instinct). I then pretty much assumed that would be my price for ever, maybe adding a bit to my hourly rate when I had kids. I didn't fully grasp commoditization and economics. Imagine this for a second: it wasn't my mindset that initially broke through my early limitations; it was basic business and commoditization that led me on a path to realizing that the majority of thoughts or 'beliefs' I had – about not only what I was capable of charging, but also what I was actually capable of on a larger scale – were completely false.

The first step to recognizing and overcoming this way of thinking occurred early one Saturday morning. I was at the train station on my way in to London to go to a seminar about how to actually run a personal-training business. I got the 6 a.m. train from Ascot in Berkshire. I would usually be asleep at that time, as I didn't work at weekends. However. on the platform I had a strange and delightful buzz. I knew I would be going to develop my business, while other trainers either had the day off or had clients. I was on my way to learn from the best and I was in the mindset of the long game, not the lie-in. To this day, it remains one of the most important days of my life.

It was at this seminar that I first realized my personal-training hours should be charged out like an airline charging for seats: at the outset they need to fill the plane, which they do by offering competitive rates.

However, as the plane begins to fill, they have what is known as demand, and the more demand there is, the more they can increase the prices. So, my way of 'limiting my seats' was to reduce my hours on the floor, and by limiting them to thirty hours of PT (six each day), I commoditized my role as a trainer.*

Every time I hit thirty hours, I put my rates up by £5 an hour. That was it! I didn't have to challenge my 'self-worth' or go on an ayahuasca retreat to find myself. It was basic business. To the question *'James why is your rate increasing?'* I'd happily say, 'I am doing too many hours,' and no one could argue with that. I did have one client who refused to pay the increase (he was a bit of a wanker), but I then said to him, 'OK, how about we do forty-five-minute sessions and you can do your own warm-up for the first fifteen minutes?' We shook hands and we both took a win from the stand-off.

I soon learned that I was earning more money from not doing any more work. Within just a few months, I was the highest-paid PT in my gym, which was ballsy, as I soon overtook one who had been training for a decade longer than I had. I was only at the sixteen-month mark when I made that change. Being better paid meant I could be more selective with clients, and before I knew it I was earning more money while having to deliver only twenty-five hours a week of personal training.

This meant I could utilize my spare time for development, so I was doing twenty-five sessions a week, finishing each day at 2 p.m., then,

---

* In fitness we have progressive overload, a quantifiable way to progress with training. But it's not just limited to adding weight. You could do slower reps, add a quarter into the movement, even pausing at the bottom of the rep – these are all ways to progress. In business, I realized that there are many ways to skin a cat also. For instance, I don't always have to raise prices, but instead I could shorten my sessions and do less time for the same money. There are so many different ways to run a business.

after studying, I'd do a little article, chat to my mum over a cup of coffee and a biscuit and have a nap before rugby training. Strangely, by doing less you can sometimes do a lot more. Going into the gym for four sessions as opposed to six or seven meant I was more inclined to put on a podcast on the drive home and I'd have the cognitive energy to remember what I heard.

The more I develop myself, the more I feel like I am paying into development which really enables me to appreciate my own self-worth. Charging more for your services is easier when you pay more into your abilities. Being tired and overworked, moving sideways and not forwards can leave you feeling like a fraud and that your services aren't worth what you have charged. I am sure any personal trainers reading this will know how it feels to deliver your eleventh session for the day and feel inclined to offer a refund to the client as they leave the facility.

If you only focus on income, you can neglect personal development and self-help. **It's funny how you can neglect your full potential and you can neglect your business at the same time by trying too hard to build it in the first place.** It's almost an effort paradox. For me, I was charging and earning nearly double what I'd ever thought I was capable of, but it wasn't what I was capable of – it was merely *what I believed* I was capable of. The boundary between what I charged and what I could charge was an invisible barrier, and I hadn't known until that point that it existed. It was a limiting belief imposed by nothing other than the environment I had subjected myself to and my belief that it was true. Little did I realize the profound impact that would have over the next few years.

I sometimes wonder whether or not a particular belief I have would hold up in a court of law. For instance, imagine this:

'Your honour, James Smith here believes no one in the world would pay him more than £100 for an hour; his evidence is what *he believes*.'

The jury and judge would laugh at me, as I'd have nothing to back up my belief, therefore it would be false and should not be a factor in making any decisions. I put this to you as a task.

> **TASK**
>
> Think of something that is holding you back now. Is it true? Is it really true? Write it down, make it real and ask yourself if it could stand up in court. That thing you're scared of – is there anything really that could prevent you from doing it? Because I very much doubt it. It's up to you to prove yourself wrong.

If you're self-employed and you're scared to charge more money for any reason, here's a nugget to help you get over the line, and your first victory could be just like mine. If you're not self-employed, keep this in mind for when you ask for your next pay rise, or you could have this very discussion with a good friend and change their entire approach to business.

INCREASING YOUR MARGINS WITHOUT INCREASING COSTS

Your (or their) business currently costs (x) amount to run. Rent, petrol, your time and whatever other expenses – consider all of that (x). What you earn is (y). Now subtract (x) from (y), and what you're left with is your 'take home' (z), right?

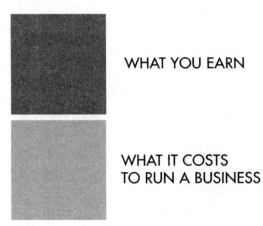

WHAT YOU EARN

WHAT IT COSTS
TO RUN A BUSINESS

You can be certain you'll be subjected to some tax, but let's ignore that for a second. If you added 10 per cent to your hourly rate, you'd expect a marginal take-home increase of simply 10 per cent, right? I thought the same, but I was wrong. Most self-employed businesses can have costs (x) which often consist of nearly half of their take home (z). So a 10 per cent increase in your rate for your client can mean a 20–30 per cent increase in your (z) margin because your costs (x) remain the same no matter how much more you charge.

*In context, this means that if your biggest fear came true and, say, 20 per cent of your clients refused to pay the higher rate, you could still go home on Thursday lunchtime for the week, take Friday off and **earn the same money**. Alternatively, if you succumbed to your limiting beliefs, without evidence, you have just reduced (y) with (x) staying the same. This means 10 per cent less earning, but a potential 20 per cent smaller take-home margin, which means working Saturday and half your Sunday for the **same money**.*

THE 10% INCREASE TO CLIENTS RESULTS IN A 20–30% MARGIN INCREASE IN TAKE HOME FOR YOU

WHAT YOU EARN

WHAT IT COSTS
TO RUN A BUSINESS

Limiting beliefs are not just financial or business related. Sure, they crop up when you don't ask for a pay rise or a promotion, but they're every-where, especially when we look at something fairly simple such as asking someone out for a drink or for their phone number. I'm sure you're all too familiar with the old *'they wouldn't be interested in me, so I'd best not say hello'*. Remember, in our imaginary court of law you'd be laughed at; and even if the worst came true, they'd just politely decline your advance by lying about having a partner already, giving a fake number or saying, 'No thanks.' Hardly going to ruin your life, is it?

Fear of Failure, Fear of Success

I never wanted a big following on social media. I never set out to be sent loads of free stuff, to host a podcast or go on national television. Some people find that hard to believe with the selfies, offers and upgrades at events. But life is not the same with a big following, I can tell you that. But like anywhere else in life where there are ups, there come consequential downs, too. Any ex-girlfriend can make up a story and go to the press with it to make a bit of cash. These days, you're just one bad tweet away from your business going under and the cancel culture will be coming for you at some point. A meaningful relationship becomes more difficult as people dress you with their own assumptions before you've even met. The more successful you become, the more perfect you're supposed to be by default.

It's meant a continual adjustment in mindset to so many areas of my life. I have, in essence, given up the majority of my privacy to enable my business to exist and my books to sell. Everything comes at a cost, but to me, social media has been imperative for any success experienced. So, what happened? Why me? And how could a number of subscribers, likes and followers actually influence my mindset about what I was able to accomplish?

Well, you see, the initial reason I created a business page was simple: to generate demand – a stream of people who liked what I had to say and who'd enquire about personal training. Like walking past a good estate agent: you see in the window a house that catches your eye, you like the location, the number of rooms and before you know it, you're enquiring about having a look around. In my case, this was an opportunity to sell myself to the person to sign up. It was quite simply about presenting a solution to a problem.

In my eyes, it means less 'walking the floor', which means fewer dreary hours spent wandering around trying to get people to become your client. Let me tell you one thing, personal trainers are insecure, so much so that we hate this aspect of our work way more than we let on. Think about this: we work so hard to look after our own bodies in a bid to eradicate our own insecurities that we make it our life's work to help others with theirs.

Any personal trainer will tell you how shit it is to talk to twenty people and then have nineteen of them politely (and often not so politely) turn you down. They do it in several ways – either with a hand gesture, a lie about how they already have a programme with another trainer or even just saying they're not interested. It was an essential part of developing a PT business and I hated every single minute of it. I spent half the day with clients who paid me what felt like way too much in relation to what I believed I was worth, then the other half making advances to gym goers who didn't want to engage in conversation. It was a bittersweet experience at both ends of a very strange spectrum, and I only ever wanted social media to be the medium that meant I could walk the floor a bit less and therefore be rejected less, too. Looking back now, I can't forget the faces people would pull when I wanted to engage in a short conversation; they'd take their headphones off and look at me as if I'd just said something offensive about their mum. I literally just wanted to say hello, introduce myself and let them know how to connect with me if they ever needed help with anything. The way I saw my social-media construct was that surely a certain percentage of my following would want to do business with me, and with a decent-sized following of a few thousand I would surely possess enough gravitas for people to think I was at least legit. So I thought, anyway.

So, in hindsight, I was insecure around rejection, but also fearful of it. I was fearful of how it could diminish and negate my self-esteem. It only takes so many rejections to want to go home with your tail between your legs. You can develop a thick skin in life, but even those with the thickest skin are affected by this fear. Before walking the floor I'd go to the bathroom, make sure I looked the part and I'd hype myself up for a few minutes before taking on the entire gym to try to book someone in for a consultation. The process became easier through repetition* (as do all processes), but the self-hype required remained the same. It's daunting every time. However, being daunted is not the only emotion you feel before having to prospect.

There is also a strange fear of success. We don't like to talk about it much either, but I believe limiting beliefs and fear of success are very much intertwined, based on a very natural, primitive emotion: vulnerability. It's human nature to not want to put ourselves in dangerous situations; it simply comes from our survival instinct or what we know as the 'fight-or-flight' response. But rather than simply avoiding physically risky situations in the way our ancestors would have done, we now also avoid emotionally 'risky' situations that could lead to embarrassment, low self-worth, shame and rejection. With my first book, *Not a Diet Book*, I often worried about it doing too well and then feeling I was exposing myself to criticism: 'What if I am wrong?' 'What if I made a big mistake with what I wrote?' 'What if people expect me to be the expert

---

* Behind mastery in any field you will always see repetition. Bruce Lee said it best with the words, 'I fear not the man who has practised 10,000 kicks once, but I fear the man who has practised one kick 10,000 times.' If you wish to get better at something, do it more.

on a subject I don't know that much about?' To fear success and to have resentment towards those who experience it around you is a contemporary cultural phenomenon.

We then fear doing well *and* not doing well. I believe we fear anything that takes us outside the norm of what we're comfortable in. Our comfort zones are guarded by these irrational fears and we must break them down if we are to leave the norm.

Imposter syndrome take II

'A fraud', 'a charlatan', misleading everyone, false success, pure luck, talking a big game and soon to be found out. The man with the clipboard will walk into the room soon and tell everyone you should not be there. Yeah, that's where I am right now writing this book.

So, when we experience success, we experience fear; we fear success. But why? Because our own minds tell us that we're imposters. I touched on this in my first book, but a lot has changed even since then, and I have more to disclose.

It's easy to feel like you're alone, but again, this is a field that has been studied in detail. There's a study on physicians from 2018 which probed them about their insecurities, self-doubt and guilt through interviews in a self-assessment manner (see References, p. 255):

Participants, even those at advanced career stages, questioned the validity of their achievements. Not all participants identified as imposters; the imposter syndrome occurred at the extreme end of a spectrum of self-doubt. Even positive feedback could not buffer participants' insecurities, which participants rarely shared with their colleagues.

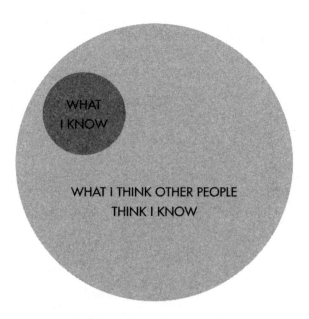

The conclusions from these studies show that it's not just the poor performers who struggle and require support, but equally those who excel in their fields. The complexities surrounding fear of success go far deeper than just imposter syndrome, but it's important we understand that it's the way our minds work.

Thoughts are much like things we walk past. **We can decide whether we engage with the emotion or the thought or whether we merely just observe it.** We only really need to know how much a rock weighs if we want to pick it up. Should we not need to pick it up, there is no need to do anything bar observe the rock for what it is: just a rock. In the same way, we can approach our emotions and feelings of being an imposter. Don't pick it up, leave it where it is, the weight is not important.

Being offended

What is it to be offended? According to the dictionary, it's to be 'resentful or annoyed, typically as a result of a perceived insult'. Stop for a second and think about how crazy it is that someone can influence our state of mind purely based on what they say. Now, this is a transactional process, although we don't see it that way – 'it takes two to tango' comes to mind. One party must say it, while the other must hear it, process it and take it to heart for it to offend them.

You can't control what happens to you in life, but you can control how you feel about it: people love to dispute this statement, but it is so true. Now, I am not saying you can stop yourself crying when your dog dies (it didn't save me when mine died). What I am saying is that we are in control of how we feel, how we react and how we handle a given situation, whether it be walking past a bakery and resisting the urge to buy something all the way to how we react to criticism.

> *Criticism is something we can avoid easily by saying nothing, doing nothing and being nothing.*
>
> Elbert Hubbard (often attributed to Aristotle)

It's normal to grieve; it's normal to get sad, to occasionally feel flat and also to be angry, frustrated – and no matter how much you decide to feel energized, if you're tired, there's no escaping it. But how we feel about what happens is more important than what happens. Of course, I could insert a cliché like 'life is 90 per cent how you react to things', but I think it's more important to address our decision to be offended in the first place. Imagine feedback – whether that's reading comments on your social-media post or hearsay from a friend's friend

– being that rock that you walk by. By enquiring about or reading those comments you are picking up the rock and taking on all of its weight. By seeking those comments out and reading them you're wanting to know the weight of the rock. **If you decide not to pick that rock up, its weight means nothing to you**, it's no longer of importance, so don't worry about it.

If I seek out criticism, I am leaving the house looking for rocks, and the further I walk, the larger the rocks I will discover. Should I decide to pick them all up, I will soon find one that I just can't pick up and it will feel like failure. If you want my advice on how to deal with criticism, my answer to you is: don't. Now, that may sound like a cop-out, but it's not; it's a legitimate strategy I utilize each and every day.

You are not obliged to deal with criticism; it's neither essential nor productive. There's feedback, which is important, of course, but that's a different ball game altogether. I am talking about the criticism from friends, loved ones and strangers on the Internet. I have experienced first-hand the extent to which personal trainers worry about what other PTs think of them, being the only people in the world who won't use their services. If someone is going to benefit your life through being a customer then yeah, you can listen. But listening to the criticism of people who won't benefit you, that's something you're not obliged to do – so don't. When someone delivers a rock to your doorstep, leave it there; you don't have to pick it up.

Taking the criticism as true? Your choice. Taking it to heart? Your choice. Accepting it as constructive? Your perception. You are opening the door to unhappiness, stop it. It won't come easy – like maintaining eye contact with a stranger, it takes practice. Next time you're criticized think of it this way:

I'd say with confidence that we can apply the 80/20 rule here: 80 per cent of your criticisms come from people who do not benefit your life,

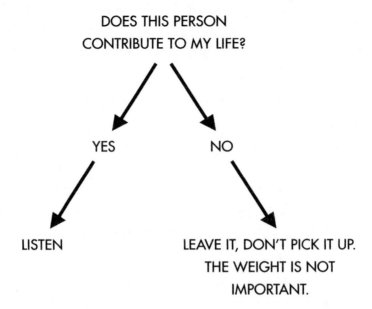

DOES THIS PERSON
CONTRIBUTE TO MY LIFE?

YES   NO

LISTEN   LEAVE IT, DON'T PICK IT UP.
THE WEIGHT IS NOT
IMPORTANT.

so, you can reduce 80 per cent of the negativity coming into your life through actually doing less. Powerful shit, right? Being offended is a self-imposed mental cruelty. It sits within the same category of those who download apps that tell you who has unfollowed you on social media – you call it curiosity, but you are proactively opening the door to things that will make you less happy. Fact. People also misinterpret being harmed and being offended. If someone punches you, that's harm. Someone defaming you or ruining a professional reputation, that's harm. Having your feelings hurt by reading your comments on social media is not harm – that's being offended, I'm afraid.

And as far as the 20 per cent of potential criticisms that come from people who do benefit your life, well, that's a place for feedback. You'll find this 20 per cent not only constructive, but when a happy customer gives you feedback, you can bet that implementing it will, more often than not, benefit how your business runs and performs.

Don't get the two confused because it's all too easy to get caught up with misidentifying them. Sometimes letting someone offend us (which is a choice) can create this turmoil inside of angst, rage and temper. We create and fabricate this burden and carry it with us, and it distracts us, annoys us, makes us tired. We carry the weight of that rock around everywhere we go. For what? For nothing. Brushing this off is not easy; simply ignoring it is a skill in itself, and I have a few ways that I deal with it.

We cannot bury emotions, we cannot click and make them disappear, but what we can do is transform them into another emotion. Criticisms create insecurities, self-doubt and despair. The despair can come from people touching a nerve because they're preying on existing insecurities. I always say that 'every joke has a small amount of truth to it'. Dismantle the next pop someone has at you and think about it. Now, don't spiral into panic just yet – I have a task for you.

TASK

For a moment, put yourself in the shoes of someone who could troll, comment and go out of their way to make a negative remark. Whether it's on your hair loss, gaining weight, looking tired or not doing a task well. Instead of getting caught up in what they said, ask yourself *why* they said it. No one says something negative for no reason; all too often, people project their own insecurities on to others. They like to spread negativity, not only to draw people down to their level, but because it's also so easy to do. We don't often even rebut people with 'neggy vibes' or negativity, largely because negative people are fucking hard to deal with – they're draining and people would rather 'let it go'

---

than have to deal with them. I think about what it must be like to be in the life of someone negative, with the glass half full, with the world against them. I think to myself for a second: the troll, the naysayer, the person who criticized me probably did it for pleasure. I think to myself: imagine if I had to resort to that to make myself happy? What a sad life and existence that would be.

When I spend just a few seconds in one of those people's shoes I no longer have angst, no longer have hatred; I'm no longer upset, deflated or negated. I feel sorry for that person instead. I reread their comment with fresh eyes and think to myself how much happiness it may have given them at the time. The rock no longer needs to picked up; by doing so I'd be giving a little bit of happiness to a very pathetic person. That person merely put a rock in my path to trip me up for their own benefit. To leave it alone and do nothing is the perfect response.

Pretend the rock isn't even there, because by deciding not to act on it, you can carry on walking unaffected.

Often those that criticize others reveal what he himself lacks.

Shannon L. Alder

TALL POPPY SYNDROME

Tall poppy syndrome is something that I first experienced in Australia during my late twenties. It is the notion that the tallest poppy is the first to be cut down.

My efforts to build an online presence were not well met when I started personal training in Australia. (I can only imagine that the repercussions of being exposed to that at an earlier stage could have potentially negatively impacted my trajectory within my work life.)

In hindsight, my poor behaviour at school protected me in some respects, as I was always told I had 'more potential' and that I was hanging around with the wrong people. I grew up hearing that I should and could accomplish more; looking back, I must have listened to them more than I realized. On the flip side, if I'd been brought up being told I couldn't accomplish anything, that I shouldn't take risks because they wouldn't pay off, I would definitely have played it safe when the opportunity presented itself, as it did later on in life.

Power plays are not limited to the chessboard and you must look out for them in both personal and professional relationships. Remember, a frog will immediately jump out of hot water, but if you heat cold water slowly enough the frog won't even notice, to its own detriment, that is. A sad statistic is that many people who are victims of gaslighting don't even know it. It can occur in a business setting, through abuse of the professional hierarchy, and it is an invisible force that negates our emotional, physiological and even physical wellbeing. There are studies on gaslighting's effect on the human psyche from the early 1980s, yet it's something that the billions of humans who get into toxic relationships are still not aware of. To me, that's like humans getting into water without the knowledge that the temperature can even change.*

Just remember that genetics only go so far in life and the rest of our development is from environment, how we are brought up and how we bring those up around us. This isn't limited to parents either – you could be an uncle, an aunt, a cousin or even a brother or sister. Your every word and action can influence people more than you know. As one of my favourite quotes goes:

My earliest memories of my father are of seeing him work at his desk and realizing that he was happy. I did not know it then, but that was one of the most precious gifts a father can give his child.

Malcolm Gladwell, *Outliers: The Story of Success*

In the universe, there is matter and then non-matter; we have yin and we have yang, we have good and we have evil, we have positively charged and negatively charged. With this in mind, I like to think that on the other end of the spectrum to 'gaslighting' we should look at positive affirmations. I don't like the idea of

---

* Gaslighting is a tactic in which a person or entity, in order to gain more power, makes a victim question their reality. Anyone can be susceptible to gaslighting, especially in relationships where there is an unequal power dynamic. It's the act of undermining another person's reality by denying facts and the environment around them, even their feelings. Victims of gaslighting are manipulated into turning against their own cognition, their emotions, and who they feel they are as a person.

'being nice for the sake of being nice'. I think that false niceties can dilute the essence of how we communicate with each other. Instead, we should look at the positive things we say as vehicles to lift those around us to become the tallest poppy, rather than wishing to cut them down. Seeing people (or poppies) taller than you should only inspire you to do more. I think putting someone down to raise your own standard is pathetic, and anything that can negatively affect someone's mental health should be eradicated from society. If you're ever worried about someone potentially having a pop at any relative success you're experiencing, just remember:

You never get put down by people above you in life.

I like to imagine an ideal whereby we all help each other, we all lift one another and give helping hands to other people with their professional and personal relationships and ambitions. When we see people do well, we have two options in my eyes: to be bitter about it or to recognize their success and up our own game in response.

The invisible game

For several years, I have been in competition with people who don't even know we are competing. I will admit it requires finite thinking, which I don't usually advocate long term; however, for short durations it's not only fun, but hugely effective.

I never make these games a pillar of my happiness or wellbeing, only a strategic ploy from time to time to feed, yes, my ego, but also the competitive inner part of me. I grew up playing video games and sports, and while you can't approach life in the way you would a video game, you can approach 'the invisible game' in the same way. When I was twenty-seven, I had a moment when I really had an honest word with myself. I said, 'James, you're not going to be the most intelligent personal trainer, nor in the best condition, nor the most experienced, nor the most popular.' There was one thing I thought I could do, though. I truly believed I could be one of the best PTs in the world at communicating. So instead of trying to get really lean or really muscular, I decided to position myself in the industry as a disruptor to speak out, to communicate and to hit home with salient points each and every day.

Just after I got my first taste of what I could call 'traction' in my mind, I turned the entire process into a game. Doing this can remove me from the task, almost like gaming in my spare time in a bid to de-stress, except in these instances I could enjoy the gaming experience within my field of work. I know a lot of adults use gaming to escape reality, but to me it was a means of making the most of reality, too.

I've never told anyone this before, but I made a list of the top ten people in my field, then week on week monitored my engagement on Facebook in comparison to theirs. These personal trainers were not only unaware that I was in competition with them, they didn't even know I existed, let alone that they were a part of my game. This was about me. It was about my growth, it was about growing my own 'poppy', and it was never about cutting anyone else's down. It was a game to grow myself; to me, the others were above me and I didn't feel bitter. I felt motivated looking up at them. One of my best friends, Lucy Lord, baked me a cake when I surpassed the first one on the list, putting me at that point at number 10. We sat back and spoke about eyeing up the next on the list and I laughed to myself as I said, 'They won't even see me coming.'

I sometimes use the same game to look at people who are just emerging in my industry. Imagining scenarios of them competing with me in my field keeps me motivated, keeps me hungry, keeps my grasp on humility. This can be done anywhere – with friends, rival businesses – and the best thing I find about no one knowing about your game is that you can decide on the rules, and there can always be a new 'competitor' once you've surpassed the previous one in the cross hairs.

I also like removing myself completely from my work sometimes and seeing it as a game instead: getting out of bed when the alarm goes off to secure the first points of the day, when everyone else snoozes and I am up and about; checking my emails during down time secures me a few more. I may be tired, I may just want to watch Netflix, but there's a primal urge to win today – to win the game and to be in the top position. **Although the idea of being in a game is finite, I have intentionally not set a position where I can actually win.** I often say that comparison is the thief of joy, and I still stand by this – but the game is not about comparison. I am not seeking external gratification. I'm simply harnessing my hunger to push the boundaries of my own markers for success. No one is in my game apart from me, no one knows about it apart from me, and when I reach the summit, I will seek a bigger and higher one. The summits will increase in height for ever because **becoming is better than being, right?**

TASK

Whether you sell used motorcycle parts, operate a plumbing business or currently have an office-based job, ask yourself what elements of your work and life could you gamify? It could even be a self-development gamification. It could be about reading ten pages before bed; it could be about learning a new language or anything you put your mind to. You can remove yourself from the task and play an invisible game, securing points. You can decide the rules and no one even needs to know the game exists. I find my life seems a lot less daunting and stressful when I see it simply as a game where I aspire to get a higher score each day.

Sometimes reading at least ten pages a day or listening to ten minutes of an audiobook/podcast is great, but if you're like me, you'll enjoy it that bit more knowing your competition won't be. Write some of your goals or objectives down, make them real. They say that 'the fox climbing the hill is always more hungry than the fox at the top of the hill'. I think about that most days. My hill has changed a lot over the past few years. In fact, right now it's bigger than ever and I wouldn't change that for anything else in the world. Your take-home from that? Stay hungry, always.

Exponential return

I love telling people that if they had only one penny and doubled it, and then doubled that again the next day, and the next and so on, before a month had passed, they'd be a multimillionaire. Writing this book, for instance: all it took was for me to type words followed by more words. That sounds like I am doing myself a disservice, but it's true. Writing words for thirty minutes each day is not impressive. It's not. However, being consistent and doing that for a few months? That's more impressive, right? Now, if you partner that with the fact that I posted on social media, well again, anyone can do that. Who doesn't have social media? Who doesn't have email? So, again, what I did was not impressive. But with consistency, I changed that. I've sent emails through marketing campaigns for years – easily six years, sending an email each day. So spending twenty minutes writing an email – that's not impressive. But sending them every day on an interesting subject is. Putting five minutes aside for a social-media post, again, not impressive. But thousands upon thousands of posts and videos and engaging with my following online and in real life cultivates the brand I live and breathe each day.

When you take the cultivation of the small posts and short emails and plot that across a graph, it would be easy to draw the conclusion that the growth was slow. But, just like the spread of COVID-19, the simple concept of exponential growth means that what seemed very little before, like that first penny, can soon equate to millions and millions of pounds.

The point I want to make clear is that wins in life rarely come from big events or big things – instead it's all about the accumulation of what would be deemed 'small steps'. To expect instant gratification also disregards how exponential growth works, and this is why you can't expect a return from your efforts right away. Exponential growth at first is hard to understand because it looks almost unimpressive. A bit like me sitting in a café in the UK writing a blog on potato vs sweet potato. It's only when you start to see your efforts, the people who read your posts and then their friends tell their friends that you realise what exponential really is.

If you'd looked at my efforts after a year, it'd be so easy to say it wasn't worth it. I had made no money or business from social media. Year 2 the same. However, a handful of years later I became a *Sunday Times* bestselling author from typing for thirty minutes a day and repeating a few times.

> On this team we fight for that inch. On this team we tear ourselves and everyone else around us to pieces for that inch. We claw with our fingernails for that inch. Because we know when we add up all those inches that's gonna make the fucking difference between winning and losing, between living and dying!
>
> *Any Given Sunday*

How many times have you put in the effort to only give up? It's so easy to give up because you look at what you have, what it looks like compared to what you see others have. But you can't get caught up with merely where you are; instead, look ahead to where it could take you. The biggest danger is to compare where you are to someone else's trajectory. Please don't forget that. **Your current trajectory is much more important than where you are right now.** So, keep doubling, keep your blinkers on, play the game, stay hungry, stay on the hill – and one day, you'll look back and wonder how you got so far ahead.

Motivation

People say they need to be motivated. I'm not sure I agree. I mean sure, I am motivated by some things in life: making people around me proud, being able to feed my primal instinct to provide for people and, of course, money – to a certain extent. I spoke about real wealth and how it's different from being financially 'rich on paper' earlier in this book. What motivates us will be governed a lot by our values, but what can we really do to remain motivated all the time?

I believe that our focus relies too much on motivation when it should be directed towards identifying things that demotivate us. That's right, we must identify all those things that derail our progress and knock us off track. For many years as a personal trainer I identified things that were demotivating people. I then set to work with those people to eradicate the habits or actions in question, and suddenly, the prospect of needing to be motivated didn't seem to be necessary.

People may not intentionally demotivate themselves, but that doesn't mean they don't do it – each and every day. I've always used the analogy of banking when it comes to someone's calorie intake: pragmatically, we don't generally aspire to put the most money away possible because we like to enjoy ourselves but remain smart. When it comes to managing food intake, however, people live on a continuum of extreme and non-existent dieting and when they run out of the motivation to continue, they sit back and think they need to be motivated. Instead of being the all-knowing guru that so many pretend to be, I like to simply show people they're not broken, just sometimes a bit foolish with their idealism.

When people are made to feel like they need motivation, they stop in their tracks. They slow their progress to a halt and they seek external intervention from someone who, in my eyes, is not only unnecessary but potentially also a charlatan (like 'life coaches' – hence the nuanced title of this book). There is every chance you may need a coach – someone to study under, someone to look up to and someone whose experiences you can learn from – but not, I think, for motivation.

I think we're all wired to want to do well. I mean that on a primal level, we all want to do the same things and we like the same luxuries, but we're all brought up influenced by slightly different values. What if I told you that those with 'self-motivating' traits are the sensible ones? What if I told you that those who need motivation are potentially the ones who are trying to accomplish too much in one go, too influenced by external factors, social media and what the person next to them is doing, rather than looking at what they already have. For years I have adopted a 'blinkers on' mentality to my work, whereby I'm focused on my own metrics, my own business and my own progress. To compare my own to someone else's isn't productive and could achieve the complete opposite to motivation. I've been crass about it before when I've said that I don't look at other men's genitals in the urinals for two reasons: for one thing, I'm pee shy, so I usually use a cubicle; and second, it's not going to change the size of my own genitals, so why look? Why compare? Why look at anyone's other than my own?

When you feel demotivated, it's important not to stop, not to wait for help, but instead to try to identify why. What is it that you're stuck with? Is it lack of progress or is it about your idea of what progress looks like and how it feels? Are you tripping yourself up? Are you being your own worst enemy in the process of trying to accomplish something?

Many individuals do not engage in health-promoting behaviours that would confer important health benefits despite research that has shown that engaging in a suite of four health behaviours (physical activity, eating a healthy diet, not smoking, and drinking alcohol in moderation) leads to a 11–14 year delay in all-cause mortality.*

For years, I've seen this with dietary change. People decide they are going to eliminate all the foods that they enjoy. They label chocolate and pizza as 'bad' and they banish them from their 'new diet'. But chocolate and pizza are not bad, let me tell you that. They're fucking fantastic – but yes, if you consume too much of either of them in relation to the amount you move around, you'll end up overweight.

So, someone is now two weeks into their 'new diet' of predominantly lean meats and vegetables. They open the fridge and don't feel the motivation to continue eating bland foods. But they know of the guilt that will come if they give in to the 'bad' foods, and they feel lost. They feel they lack willpower and they doubt they're going to be able to continue or whether the end goal is really worth it. This person could then call me up and say, 'James, I need help. I struggle to stay motivated with eating a good diet.' I have had this conversation hundreds of times, but they don't need me to motivate them; they actually need me to educate them on what a good diet is and that chocolate is not bad, but just has to be managed, along with the pizza, of course. When I reintroduce both foods, let's say, I then manage their expectations a bit, maybe even lengthen the timeframe for the expected outcome, and suddenly, what does that person feel? More motivated to stick to their 'new diet'. Now, did I give that person motivation or did I remove their own recurrent demotivators?

* See References, p. 255.

The conversation could be the same with someone who is expecting their tech start-up to sky rocket in its first year, or their child to be the best behaved in their school or who keeps getting tapped out in each session of jiu jitsu. The issue is all too often rooted in expectations, not levels of motivation. People get in their own way; they just don't always see it clearly.

I feel very strongly that we should use this thinking with the obese, for instance: rather than offering them money or incentives to lose weight, we must realize that they're already motivated. Not many obese people wake up wanting to be obese – of course they want to lose weight, but they have a string of failed attempts behind them, no doubt accompanied by unsustainable objectives and the influence of social factors, and because of this, many of them consistently engage in bad habits and feel they need motivation, when what they really need is new and better daily habits.

Author James Clear says it best when he says that a mistake only happens once. If it happens again, it's no longer a mistake but the beginning of a bad new habit; develop enough of those and they begin to construct your identity.

Forming good habits is an integral part of not needing to rely on seeking motivation to do things, a bit like making your bed: what may have felt like a chore at first becomes a part of your identity – once you have done it enough times you no longer need to be motivated to do it; through repetition you've made it intrinsic. All too often, people decide to identify as someone who 'lacks motivation'. Little do they know they usually just set poor goals to accomplish, a constant flow of things to trip themselves up on their desired route.

Qualifications

Some people love to learn, and this chapter is not an attack on them. It is more to do with those who use qualifications as something to hide behind. You know who you are! You use qualifications as somewhere to put your efforts, and rather than it being about *the level of qualification*, it's the level of self-worth you seek.

Believe it or not, a qualification is also a belief system that consists of no matter: it cannot be touched or quantified outside of learnt human behaviour. You can spend years and thousands of pounds to attain a qualification. It can get you jobs, prevent you from getting others and people will judge you on your grade, your level of attainment.

There are a lot of roles which I am very glad call for qualifications, don't get me wrong. Pilots, doctors, accountants, nurses, etc. However, for many outside of those professions, they are a way to amplify their own self-worth, not just to themselves, but to others, too.

I can't help but feel that people lose sight of important values and would rather be the most qualified in the room than the best at the job in question. In my experience of personal training, I've seen those who are the best coaches and those who are the best qualified. There is often not much of a correlation between the two. You can be a well-qualified but dog-shit coach. On the flip side, you can be poorly qualified on paper but a great coach in practice.

Those of a scholarly nature tend to remain within the academic scene and sometimes sheltered from the real world. Grades become degrees which become Masters which become PhDs which become second PhDs. Some are pursuing a passion, but others are chasing qualifications that will allow them to have sufficient self-worth to believe in themselves. This can take years, even decades, and there is no guarantee that they will ever get that elusive feeling.

I find that some people use their qualifications and accolades as a part of their identity. It's apparent from the outside looking in that for a lot of them it's a badge of honour they like to wear. For me, I would much rather let my work demonstrate my ability. I've studied on courses and not taken the exams, and people think that's crazy, but to me it's not. The reason I am this way inclined is I that don't think people should study for grades. They should study for some of the most valuable commodities in the real world, namely confidence and self-worth.

So, if you're well qualified, that's great. But if you're not, do not let that hold you back. It's a belief system; it cannot be touched or felt, it can only be printed on paper. If you are great at something, then believe in your ability to do it. On paper, I am one of the least qualified personal trainers in the world. I got the essential qualifications required to legally do my job, but the rest I did myself. I have no qualifications in marketing, social media, video editing, communications or PR. But I've never let that become a barrier between me and the people I wish to help. I failed both my English qualifications at GCSE level, but here I am on my second book without a sniff of a ghost writer at hand.

The Confidence Paradox

Having said all of the above, I can appreciate that a qualification may amplify confidence for some. Take this scenario, for instance: when you pass your driving test you're only forty minutes more experienced as a driver, but once you've got the nod and you've passed, you feel uplifted and more confident – you're no longer a learner and your status has changed. You hit the road a new person. How can such a small shift in experience and a qualification in itself have such a profound impact?

It's about belief: someone else believes in you and that is something powerful. The driving instructor is backing your ability in the form of passing you. But to me, it's equally important that we believe in ourselves. Confidence is such a powerful tool, yet we're never taught about it in school. Confidence is a secret weapon and if you master it, you can get paid better, get laid more often and succeed in whatever you want in life. I know it sounds clichéd, but we can't sit around and wait for people to instil a sense of confidence in us like we would when learning to drive. It's an internal battle, an internal dialogue and a daily fight with our own protective mechanisms within our heads.

> Confidence is a state of being clear headed either that a hypothesis or prediction is correct or that a chosen course of action is the best or most effective. Confidence comes from a Latin word 'fidere' which means 'to trust'; therefore, having self-confidence is having trust in one's self.*

* See References, p. 255.

Confidence isn't just about what you say; it's how you say it, your body language, your course of action and how you present or market yourself in every moment. It begins with self-belief and again, you can't buy self-belief or top it up overnight – it comes from your identity and how you perceive yourself. Many people play into the idealism of 'fake it till you make it' but unfortunately that's about as helpful as shouting 'calorie deficit' to an obese person or 'cheer up' to a depressed person.

I see confidence as a skill, just like learning to do a snatch in Olympic lifting or practising a golf shot. You must be overzealous at times and **a degree of audacity is imperative**. Carry yourself tall, walk with your chest out, shoulders back and don't worry about being wrong. Practise confidence; hold people's gaze and don't be afraid to wait until they look away first.

Imagine confidence as a fabric; you must stretch it or it will stay the same. It takes repetition, too: the more frequently you stretch the fabric, the more you will grow. There are no rules as to the elasticity of this fabric. The way it acts is not governed by physics and there is no fixed amount of strength required to pull on it. I'll speak about worst-case scenarios in the following chapter, but at every opportunity we should look to stretch the fabric, not too fast, but at the right rate. A stand-up comedian stretches theirs at the small venues, repeating the same jokes, night in, night out, building up to the grand tour in front of thousands in an arena. You see a comedian without fear, oozing confidence, but you don't see the hours of practice when they stretched their own fabric through repetition. We're exposed to and experience other people's confidence and we think that they're born with it (or that they're great pretenders), but behind every skill set is repetition. The fabric of confidence is within our imagination and it plays to no rules. The rate at which you stretch it is governed by you and you alone. If you get nervous speaking in front of only a few people, I'm here to tell you that speaking in front of thousands would only be blocked by any feelings you choose to feel about it. You're more than capable of doing it, you just need to tear down the self-imposed rules that you've created in your head to stop any stretching of the 'fabric of confidence'.

Some people interestingly think that standing in a toilet cubicle with your hands over your head as a power pose before a big event is going to increase your confidence tenfold, but I think that attitude does a huge disservice to the small battles won each day on the way to becoming the confident person who wins the job interview.

Without stetching the 'give' of the fabric of confidence, it will stay the same. Fitness is all about pushing boundaries to evolve performance, incremental increases over time with progressive forms of overload. It sounds oversimplified, but some people stretch their fabric and many others don't. If you're not willing to push your boundaries no power pose is coming to save you. This is on you and how you act from the turn of this page all the way up until the day you're no longer able to turn a page. Morbid, I know, but it's coming, so don't wait around.

Stretching the fabric: self-worth

Self-esteem is an individual's subjective evaluation of their own worth. Self-esteem encompasses beliefs about oneself (for example, 'I am unloved', 'I am worthy') as well as emotional states, such as triumph, despair, pride and shame.*

* See References, p. 255.

Jump on to Instagram and it's not long before you find a picture of someone in perfectly acceptable shape pinching their fat with a caption that mentions something to do with self-esteem, self-compassion, self-acceptance, self-respect, self-confidence, self-love and self-care. What on earth are people talking about?

It's how we feel about ourselves, simply. But I want to broaden the scope of this topic here to more than just how we look with our tops off. Ultimately, feeling worse about ourselves is profitable. Think about it: from anti-wrinkle cream to falling behind on fashion trends or not being in good enough shape to fit in with a perceived norm. If we have poor self-esteem, we'll make very good consumers.

It's not easy, however, to communicate with our emotions or to get an accurate gauge on where we are at. **Self-worth and self-esteem are the foundations of our mental health, just as sleep and nutrition are the foundations of our fitness or 'wellbeing' regimes.** But self-esteem is not a fabric that can be stretched like confidence – you can't count to three and step outside your zone like you can with confidence-building exercises. And there are ample links between poor self-esteem and depression. (See References, p. 255.)

So, what determines our self-esteem? Interestingly, this ties in closely with our values and is defined as net worth for many people. How much they're worth is usually based upon their place within a social hierarchy, which is fed by income, material possessions or the acquisition of as many assets as possible, like a financial monopoly.

Who you know and your social circle can have big impacts on your perception of your self-worth. Some people can rate their status on who they know, who's important and what influence they have. Some people think the reason for the growing selfie culture is that posting a picture with someone of influence or fame can raise their perceived status. I've yet to find a study on celebrity selfies, but people taking pictures of themselves to fulfil basic human needs like popularity and self-expression is a well-researched area, showing that it makes people feel better about themselves.

What you do is often a big factor in self-esteem, and this is hugely influenced by culture, but there's often a stigma with certain professions (such as teaching, although hugely important for the development of future generations), while some may consider a doctor or banker to be at a more important professional level. What you achieve is also a big player in self-esteem; for some people, being the most qualified in the room is of the utmost importance in improving their self-esteem and therefore perceived self-worth.

Then there's appearance. Although one of the more relevant factors, I have left this till the end, as it ties into the next part of the book. We all know about the peculiar obsession with how much we weigh. Most of the world's popular weighing clubs build a business model around it. And I can quote from *Not a Diet Book*, where I said, 'Your self-worth cannot be quantified by your relationship to gravity.' Weight fluctuates not solely according to our success or our efforts, but so many other factors from, yes, fat loss to bowel movements, hydration and where you are on your menstrual cycle (for half of us, anyway). Clothing sizes are also a big thing, more so for women, and there's even stigma surrounding certain sizes.

One of the biggest factors surrounding our self-worth and how much store we place on our appearance is what happens, for example, when someone flirts with us, asks us out or we hear a murmur that someone finds us attractive. This has a huge beneficial impact on our self-esteem – much greater than any arbitrary weight loss or a drop in clothing size. Losing a few pounds is one thing, but having three attractive people ask for your number in one week? I know which I'd pick.

I have drawn many conclusions from modern-day social media and its diminishing effect on self-esteem, but what do you think about this for a hypothesis: are we relying so much on dating apps that we're damaging our ability to boost each other's self-esteem by no longer approaching people, flirting or asking anyone out? Which brings me to a very interesting point where we could bring two elements together and think about the potential outcome for confidence and self-esteem, or the 'worst-case scenario'.

Worst-case scenario: Stretching the fabric in practice

That's it. Ask yourself that, all the time.

Let me tell you this: I have over a million followers, a TED Talk, a best-selling book and a multi-million-dollar revenue online business. You'd think I'd have the confidence to ask a stranger for their number, but lo and behold, I still shit my pants every time. Every time. Suddenly, my mind will be racing with thoughts, most of which I have no evidence to back up when I challenge them: she's probably married and not wearing her wedding ring; probably got a boyfriend who is going to get super angry and beat me up from behind … Your mind fills with fear and anxiety, your heart rate increases and your palms begin to sweat. I make up all these wild excuses – every excuse possible – to not make an approach: maybe next time, this doesn't feel right, she will see I'm nervous, what if she doesn't speak English?

Then my inner pragmatist pipes up: 'James, what is the worst that can happen here? Like actually the worst? Let's say I go over: "Hello, I think you're really attractive and I would love to take you for a drink. Here's my number if you're keen."'

Scenario 1: 'I'm really sorry, I have a boyfriend.' Whether true or not it's a kind decline. We never know circumstances, so we can't produce our own to fit the agenda.

Scenario 2: 'Sure.' But then she never texts me. OK, cool. Is this really a bad thing? With email marketing, if 99 per cent of my email list do not buy from me, I still have a very successful campaign. With one in a hundred buying my cheapest product, let's say, on a list of 260,000 people (which it is at current), that's £23,300 (42,514 AU$) from a single email. Not bad from a 99 per cent failure rate.

Either way you look at it, it's a win. Worst-case scenario, you've complimented a stranger, perhaps making their day; best case is they say yes (even if you get ghosted down the line). Either way, you went for it – you won't be mocked, you'll be admired as a go-getter, a do-er. **In the modern world of constant distractions and technology, the simple art of talking to a stranger is dying.**

Whether we lose a job or don't get a promotion, perform poorly in a workout or break up with a loved one, I don't think we really appreciate the worst possible outcome. Going for a job that you're not quite 'experienced' enough for, you may not get a second interview, but at least you went for it. You ended up in the same position before you applied and walked away a couple of hours poorer, but that little bit more experienced in the uncomfortable situation of being interviewed. These risks compound interest in your identity. Each is an opportunity to stretch the fabric of what you are comfortable with, an opportunity not everyone will take. An opportunity to inch ahead of everyone else.

The best advice I've ever had: the silver-lining effect

What happens when things do turn out bad? I'll never forget the wise words I heard from Scott.

Scott trained at Fitness First George Street in Sydney with one of my best friends, Diren Kartal, as his coach. 'Hello, James,' he'd say in his American accent, having heard me from wherever I was on the floor. Scott was blind but still trained four times a week. (Next time you are a little bit sore and considering skipping the gym, just think of Scott, fully blind and still making more trips to the gym than most of us.) I'll never forget Scott telling Diren and me his story.

Scott sold companies to IBM and made a fortune in his early twenties only to find out at twenty-six that he had a rare eye disease and would very soon be blind and no longer able to drive the fancy Porsche he'd just bought. Scott has forever been in my mind since I met him; if I knew I only had my eyesight for a few more years, I think any financial savings would be shunted down the priorities list and I'd set my sights (pardon the pun) on seeing as much of the world as I could, so that I'd always have the memories when I was older.

The thought of a debilitating condition really prompts us into action to accomplish things we want to do. We shouldn't need to think like that, but unfortunately, it's probably our default mindset. If you were going to go blind next year, would you leave tomorrow via a myriad of dodgy cheap flights to go see the sun set over the Rocky Mountains in the USA and Canada?

I bet you'd think that Scott was pissed off. Well, he wasn't; he was one of the nicest and happiest guys I have ever met. And he gave Diren and me some of the best advice possible which has got us both out of a lot of mental sticky situations. I had in twenty-four hours not only broken up with my girlfriend who I was about to move in with, I'd also lost my visa to Australia where I was living and setting up a life. Diren had decided to exit an eight-year relationship and, well … what Scott said in one sentence changed everything.

'Guys, no matter what happens, you will be just fine.'

Now, if you're going to take some advice from someone, I'm not sure anyone is better qualified than a very intelligent, successful man who lost his eyesight through no fault of his own. I have applied his thought process to so much. Whether I tear my anterior cruciate ligament (ACL) in my knee rolling in my next jiu jitsu session, whether I get sued for speaking out against charlatans or if no one buys this book. Guess what? **I'll be just fine.**

My lawyers need bills to get by, after all; I'm sure they have mouths to feed. And during my rehab I could listen to a lot of audiobooks and study Brazilian jiu jitsu in my spare time – the amazing thing about the sport is that you can become a better athlete away from the mats, too. **A setback is only a setback if you see it that way.** A setback can be a set-up for a comeback. It's all about perception, isn't it? I could find out how my ACL went, how to prevent it happening and even raise awareness for my peers to ensure they don't make the same mistake that I did. I could even go down the rabbit hole of preventative measures and sell an ebook on it, make a shitload of money and donate the profits to pay for operations for jiu jitsu athletes who don't have private cover. The worst-case outcome from training can be effortlessly spun into a positive with just the right thinking. I can't make my knee bullet-proof any time soon, but I can alter how I see the 'worst-case scenario'. I guess the truth is that things that happen to us can only negatively impact our mental wellbeing if we let them. The worst-case scenario mindset is a choice, like so much in life.

Choose not to be harmed – and you won't feel harmed.
Don't feel harmed – and you haven't been.

Marcus Aurelius

I can't help but think that doubtful what-if thoughts of worst-case scenarios are a protective mechanism from our primitive mindset, a throwback to when the objective was to stop us falling out of trees and breaking our necks. But many of these instincts counterintuitively hold people back from doing things that can feed into the good life, such as approaching someone attractive for a date or going for an interview for a job you may like more than your current one.

This, to me, is the 'silver-lining effect'. Every single negative thing has a silver lining, a positive to it. Moving back in with the parents because I'm skint? More family time. Your dog sadly having to be put down? One less mouth to feed and to worry about until you give a new dog a perfect home. Gained a load of weight? A chance to take some time to work on you – having a lot of fat to lose is a tremendous incentive if you think about it. Just remember that our problems are only as big as we make them; they only affect us when we let them. There is a positive behind every negative, and if you seek it out, you'll find it. Also, when your problems really get on top of you, think about this:

If we could all put our problems into one big pile, we'd take
our own problems back every single time.

Lucy Lord, great friend and even better baker

It's very important that we have this approach to the worst-case scenario with our problems because – and this can be a very hard pill to swallow – we will always have problems. I've noticed that people brought up without real problems are some of the first to struggle with anxiety and sometimes depression. This isn't to say that all depressed and anxious people were brought up with a silver spoon; more that we should sometimes count our problems as a blessing.

> *Happiness is not the absence of problems,*
> *but the ability to deal with them.*
>
> Charles-Louis de Montesquieu

A single coin makes the most noise in an empty jar, so they say. Having one single problem in life I am sure makes it feel amplified. That's only normal. Another key to the good life, I suppose, is to enjoy your problems and to appreciate all the good things that come with solving them.

There's a silver lining in every problem and issue we face; we must look to find it. Again, it's up to you to choose to do so. We cannot wish for a life without problems, so I hope you understand the importance of discovering the lessons or opportunities that lie hidden within them.

PART IV
IDENTITY

Identity: condition or character as to who a person or what a thing is; the qualities, beliefs, etc. that distinguish or identify a person or thing.

I've mentioned identity several times in this book and I think it's vital to talk a bit more about what it is and why it holds such importance. As a personal trainer, you're not just educating people but actually trying to make changes in their identity. It's not always about how other people perceive them either; I think it's more important to change the way someone perceives themselves. We have the external identity which people can influence with how they dress, what they wear and how they present themselves. Whether it's 'edgy', smart or conservative, people wear an identity in some form, even down to how they do their hair and present themselves. Body language is a big player in identifying someone's traits, and just by watching someone walk, sit or engage in conversation you can find out a lot about that person.

Non-verbals are ways in which we can try to assess what someone is like. From holding eye contact to a firm handshake, we can get clues to who they are or how they want to be perceived.

I'd like to think the changes I have made to people's lives as a personal trainer are mostly identity related. For instance, taking some-one from a 'gym newbie' to a 'regular gym goer' – to me, that's an identity change. When I promote someone to hit their 10,000-step count each day, they suddenly don't just take the stairs, they become 'a person who takes the stairs'. A fit lifestyle is more of an identity than anything else; you apply that identity in the same way as your values, by living and breathing it, until it feels normal.

Here's the important thing to keep in mind: **you don't need to be someone else to improve your life**. You need to be you, perhaps even the old you. For instance, if I met you in the gym, I would not create who I wanted you to become – some idealistic notion of the perfect human. Absolutely not. Instead, I'd regress you to who you were before. For example, for many people who have had kids or an increase in workload and responsibilities, over the years they lose sight of their old identity, so it's about getting that back through instilling good habits, which is much more important than trying to mould this person into what you want them to be. If you're an alcoholic, then it's about dialling it back to when you didn't drink; if you have an issue with recreational drugs, it's not about becoming a brand new person but instead about going back to the version of you that didn't do drugs. It's important to do it this way because you've done this before: you've lived life without drinking or taking drugs before, so you know you can do it again.

Creating an identity is not about being perfect; it's about being more consistent.

I eat well, but I have days when I don't. I aspire to write marketing emails every day, but some days I am too hungover to even touch my laptop. I work hard every day, but some days I don't get a lot done. That doesn't mean I am broken, and I do not lose sleep over it. Like I said in my first book, *Not a Diet Book*: just because you get a flat tyre doesn't mean you need to get out there and slash all the others. Remember, when you fail at something more than once, it's no longer an accident but the formation of a bad habit.

When a boxer throws a combination of punches he doesn't – and can't – expect every one to be a clean hit. More often than not, when a knockout punch is thrown you will see the boxer complete the combination of punches; the brain was focused on throwing the combination much more than it was looking for a victory with each punch. See this combination as your routine and throw every punch you can, never expecting them all to hit. And don't lose sleep when you miss. Focus on repetition, practice and falling in love with the time out of the ring improving the flow, rhythm and timing. Before long it will feel natural. If you miss the same punch more than once, maybe take it back to the drawing board, as you may be now forming a bad habit. I use this boxing analogy at business seminars. Days off from marketing your business are simply times you throw no punches. Don't feel defeated; come back stronger and throw smarter.

I think walking the walk is much more important than talking the talk when it comes to identity. This is why I am always in favour of things you can instil into your identity on a daily basis, like a step count. You can, at the end of every day, have that under your belt to prove not to others but to yourself that you're an active person – you're back to your old ways of taking the stairs, not the lift. When we look to something like gym training, often life can get in the way, and whether it's our kids, our job or our energy levels that let us down, we can often feel very deflated. The reason for this is that it's not just because we missed the gym – it's that we missed the opportunity to prove to ourselves that we're now a gym goer, and with every missed session we feel a little bit of that identity being stripped away. You question who you are, how much you want it, and you can take it very personally. All it takes is two or three missed sessions in a row before you've derailed your identity and become someone 'who used to go to the gym'. This is why many people stress the importance of paying into your identity with training first thing, removing the variables that can get in the way.

Whether your goal is to be more active, more outgoing, more caring or perhaps to do more for marketing your business, think about actionable tasks or habits that you can do on a daily basis to get there. You need to remind yourself of who you are; from making your bed the second you wake up to flossing when you brush your teeth each morning – those are the little habits that make you the 'tidy person', the 'person with great gum hygiene'. Just saying you're going to get around to something isn't enough, and often, it all too easily gets put off or forgotten about altogether.

Only ideas won by walking have any value.

Friedrich Nietzsche

TASK

Walk more. It may sound silly, but you can conduct business meetings on the move; I'm sure even the person you're meeting would rather a walk than a sit down. Walking dates are a great idea. Stuck for creativity? Airplane mode ON, music or no music – and walk. If I am ever early for something, I do this: instead of sitting around for fifteen minutes, then getting an Uber, I walk the first fifteen minutes (even on a long trip) and then get an Uber from wherever I am at that point. This not only gets my steps up, but saves me money on the fare.

The active-person identity doesn't just stop at hitting more steps than others or at a commitment to a cause – there are many other layers to *just* being an active person. You can walk glued to your iPhone and seeking the next hit of dopamine or productivity. On the other hand, you can use it as a meditative practice. My best ideas come to me when I am either in the shower or when I'm out on a jog or a walk. I keep a notes section on my phone to write them down. When we are without distraction our minds do their best work.

Spanish artist Salvador Dalí* used an interesting method to come up with ideas for his work. He would fall asleep holding a spoon over a glass from a comfy position on a sofa. As he slipped into sleep, he would release the spoon, waking himself up, which gave him some incredibly vivid creative ideas for his work. Now, I am not saying that you need to do the same; what I am saying is that given the way our minds work, it's important that they're not always stimulated and distracted by our phones.

If you commit to 10,000 steps a day, 6,000 could be done and dusted during a one-hour walk; you could use it to listen to music or an audiobook, even a podcast. That's seven hours a week of learning. Not only do you become fitter, but you can learn and let your mind wander for an hour each day. And the benefits go way beyond creativity, all the way into the realm of mental health, too. You may get lost in a fiction book. I am telling you now that *The Hunger Games* was much better to read than to watch – more brutal and my imagination conjured up a much better picture than any television screen. You could get into a podcast about space or one about history; I even listened to one recently about species being discovered which we'd previously thought were extinct. There are no limits.

* Dalí is the character used on the masks in the initial season of *Money Heist* on Netflix.

Daniel Kahneman's book *Thinking, Fast and Slow* really helped me to understand how our brains tend to work when it comes to decision making. Kahneman hypothesized that our brains have two main systems. He named them System 1 and System 2.

System 1 is the fast one and it's automatic. It's effortless, by nature, and subconscious. It's why you flinch when someone grabs a hair on your top to pick it off. It's why you jump to conclusions and make judgements in an instant. Have you ever been in a scenario where you're doing a crossword with family members and you're all trying your hardest to find a word – it's a competition to see who can solve it. You say out loud, 'Erm, OK, so it's a fish, four letters.' Someone screams 'SHARK!' and you turn to them with a confused look. They then realize that you said it was four letters, but their brain had already jumped to a conclusion and just screamed it out. This is System 1. System 1 also plays a role when we forget a word; we often have to distract ourselves with another task for it to come back to us, saying, 'Hold on, it will come to me shortly.' It is when we take our minds off it that we let System 2 take control.

System 2 only handles around 2 per cent of our brainpower, leaving an astonishing 98 per cent to shout 'SHARK!' at family members. System 2 is deliberate, effortful and rational. Imagine this scenario for a second: you're walking down the street on a winter's day. You see someone in a tracksuit and their hood up walking straight towards you. Your immediate thought is that they look dodgy and you should cross the road to avoid them. The fact that they have their hood up makes you think they're trying to hide their identity and they're likely to rob you. Then, suddenly, System 2 comes in to snatch your attention with some rationality, providing ideas like, 'Well, it is cold, so the hood might be keeping their ears warm.' Whether you cross the road to avoid them or not will be a mixture of both systems working in unison, but ultimately, your brain will have created a prejudice and discriminated based on someone's appearance alone. This is the primitive brain doing what it does best: keeping us safe. It's important to note that System 2 is a slave to System 1 and that is why Dalí kept the spoon over the glass before falling asleep.

Before we move on, **if I was to say to you don't tell me what 2 + 2 equals**, you can't even help yourself. OK, how about a visual? Which of the horizontal lines below is wider? (See References, p. 255.) You have one second to answer.

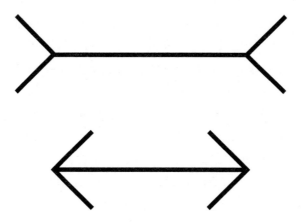

System 1 is responsible for a lot of issues that can arise due to its automatic nature, for instance jumping to conclusions. Your partner doesn't text you back and you think they could be blanking you or that you've done something wrong; System 2 then realizes they usually train in the gym this time of day, so they could be exercising. Another great example is when you learn to drive: your first dozen hours behind the wheel are very System 2; so much thought and calculation goes in to the biting point of the clutch, when to indicate and when to check mirrors. Over time, though, the cognitive effort of driving becomes System 1 through repetition.

The main reason I bring these systems to your attention is that whether the action is transitioning in yoga from Warrior II to Downward Dog or in jiu jitsu taking your opponent's back with a berimbola (fancy rolling movement), it's never without cognitive effort the first time. Only through repetition do we master a skill so that it becomes natural to us.

In jiu jitsu, there's the saying that 'drillers are killers', meaning that whoever drills a move the most will be most effective with it in sparring. In my first book, I quoted the American writer and historian Will Durant: 'We are what we repeatedly do. Excellence, therefore, is not an act, but a habit.' That's because you're moving things from System 2 to System 1. I hope that having read this chapter you'll achieve two things:

1. An appreciation that something as simple as walking with some music or a podcast is powerful far beyond just exercise; it's a means of letting your mind wander, to let System 2 do its thing. Although your System 1 brain wants to swipe Instagram, it's not to your advantage. Do your steps – after all, as Nietzsche and I agree, some of your best ideas are to come by doing so.

2. When you learn to drive, the experience is overwhelming because it feels like that there are far too many things to juggle, but over time you master them all fine. Apply that to other areas of your life: whether it's a complex lift or a skill you are seeking to improve, repetition will soon take tasks on the journey from cognitive to automated, like typing on a keyboard, for instance.

Instead of the overwhelming feelings you can experience with learning a new skill, a new hobby or whatever it is, just take a deep breath and remember that all of us work in the same way and we experience the same troubles. It will get easier and you will become better. Just give it time, give it repetition.

Perception

Perception is powerful, a big contributor to modern-day self-esteem issues; it also massively impacts how we feel about our current situation, our current state of success and where we're at (or not at) in life.

Perception: the way in which something is regarded, understood or interpreted.

I'm sure if you were to hang around a basketball team, you'd feel short. If you were to hang around fitness enthusiasts, you'd feel lazy and if you were to hang around with models, you'd feel unattractive.

I think the contrast effect comes into play more than we realize, and social media drives and fuels this, in more cases than not literally fucking us up. There are many purported benefits to social media and the Internet. However, on the flip side, they have opened a huge door to inadequacies, poor self-esteem and dissatisfaction – largely just through people's perception.

Perception can be changed in an instant, as with the yacht analogy earlier (see p. xv). At a cost of millions of pounds, you could sail for thousands of miles, only to turn up next to a bigger and better yacht, making you feel completely different about your own, and it would be difficult to shake that experience.

I have spent much of my career as a personal trainer realigning people with better perceptions of themselves and others. In a world where we compare our behind-the-scenes reality to people's high-lights reels, it's important to know that fitness models are the million-aires of the fitness industry. Being a millionaire doesn't mean you're by default happier, it doesn't mean you have a simpler life and often, behind the scenes, there are many downsides. I like to change people's perceptions of what a lot of the fitness industry really is: hungry people with a huge abundance of external pressure to look a certain way. Imagine being out of a job for gaining weight? Imagine the pressure of worrying about a fitter, younger version of you coming along any day or having to sell a certain quota of supplements month on month to pay for your rent that you're struggling to afford.

By aligning people with the real world and a different perception I can get them to feel better about not only where they are going, but where they are now – this is all without making any practical changes, simply by resetting their mindset. The power of that is massive. **In an hour, you cannot make someone more muscular or noticeably leaner, but you can make them *feel* better.** Not only that, but you can also give them a new relationship with aspects of their life that could be draining their energy and stealing from their self-esteem. Mental health, confidence and how we feel about ourselves balance so delicately on our perception of our surroundings, which is why it is so important.

We follow the richest, fittest and most popular people on the planet, and if you think your subconscious isn't making comparisons behind closed doors, you're usually wrong. How many people do you know who own a Lamborghini? Yet how many have you seen on social media? How many of your friends really have a six-pack? How many have you seen on social media? See where I'm going with this?

What we're exposed to – and what we expose ourselves to – is pushing us down, numbing us to believe we're not capable of achieving what others are and therefore creating a generation of people in a fixed mindset, not wanting to learn, develop or be inspired and instead just consuming and looking to be entertained.

> **TASK**
>
> Try taking a walk with your phone in your pocket, no music, nothing. Just walk and think. Wait until you have the urge to put your hand in your pocket; before you know it you're on your phone swiping needlessly on social media. If you want to really play a trick with your brain, move an app, even just one space away from where it normally is, and see how many times your finger goes back there without thinking. Like turning up at the fridge door increasingly often when you're not even hungry.

Introducing dopamine

Dopamine is a neurotransmitter. Think of it as a chemical messenger, playing a big role in mood, learning, motivation, heart rate and sleep. Drugs like cocaine are notorious for offering a big hit of dopamine. Sugar gets a rep for being 'just like cocaine'; however, I think that's a bit excessive. I don't think you'd find many people sharing a cubicle in a nightclub to get a hit of Fruit Pastilles.

This is not to downplay the severity of dopamine's influence within social media. Some experts even go as far as to say that it's breaking down and destroying how society works. I think society will have to adapt to social media, though, as I don't see it going away any time soon. What you'll have noticed in the task where you felt the urge to check your social media was what's known as a 'short-term dopamine feedback loop', and experts will say that this social-media issue is becoming a bona fide addiction. But before you consider going cold turkey, I found a study (see References, p. 255) on the psychological impact of a seventy-two hour withdrawal from smartphones.

> The results revealed that being restricted from one's smartphone causes more negative effects compared to not being restricted. Furthermore, spurred by the restriction, higher levels of smartphone addiction elicited more withdrawal-related symptoms.

So, on average a smartphone user can experience over 2,500 touches a day, over two hours of use each day, which isn't so much a bad thing, but it's certainly something to be aware of. In 2018, the 'screen time' feature on iOS was introduced in a bid to raise awareness of our usage, and again, what gets measured gets improved – so quantifying our time on phones could benefit people's situations should they use it too much.

But what is too much? Everything is about the dose, if you ask me. Drinking, all in the dose: too much and you'll be hungover. Doughnuts? Amazing, but eat too many for the amount you move around each day and you'll gain body fat. What is too much smartphone usage? Well, this is something that's being studied at the moment, and worryingly, high usage can be linked with poor sleep and an overall negative effect on your mental health (see References, p. 255):

Depression, anxiety, and daytime dysfunction scores were higher in the high smartphone use group than in the low smartphone use group. Positive correlations were found between the Smartphone Addiction Scale scores and depression levels, anxiety levels, and some sleep quality scores.

There is a growing body of evidence which associates too much time on your smartphone with increased chances of developing depression. My hypothesis on this is that in a world where we seek gratification, likes, follows and dopamine hits from social media, we could be left not seeking that same reward response in everyday life from social occasions, meaningful relationships or pursuing challenges within, say, fitness or in the gym.

Note: it's important that I make this clear, too: there is also a growing body of evidence for a correlation between phone use while driving and fatal car accidents. While we're on the topic, it goes without saying that you should not seek dopamine hits from your phone while driving. A no-phone-while-driving policy could not only save your life, but others', too.

People crave distractions from their current lifestyle, rather than inspiration to develop it. Development seems like something that is a turn-off for the brain, but all your best skills were learned and developed. Learning to skateboard to me was about development, and to this day it remains one of my favourite things to do. At twenty-seven, I lived a bit of an awkward distance from the beach (about a fifteen-minute walk), so I found myself sometimes wondering whether it was worth it for a dip. But I came to realize that as I lived at the top of the hill, I could probably skateboard down it in five minutes.

I went to a shop that sold skateboards. Having never been on one before, I said to the assistant, 'Mate, how do I slow down on it?' He looked at me baffled, and I said, 'Don't worry', as I felt embarrassed that I'd asked a daft question. I spent the next year of my life covered in cuts and bruises – my elbows, knees and even my shoulders became constant sites for grazes. At twenty-eight, I felt like I had my life together, but one pothole can substantially change your circum-stances, let me tell you that.

I love telling people about this because they often say, 'I couldn't do that' (limiting belief) or, 'My co-ordination is terrible' (skill not repeated enough yet), which could, in fact, be true. But co-ordination is learned and, yes, developed. No one is born with the ability to walk on a tight-rope; it's a skill, like everything else. So much is learned from the first time you fall off – again, like failure in life, the first stack should be embraced. Without it you won't develop.

I give lessons to my friends on how to skateboard. I always say, 'So, *when* you fall off' (never *'if'*), as it's all about when it's going to happen. It's inevitable. Even now, as a pretty decent skater, I know that I just fall off a lot less than I used to. As I develop, my chances of falling off decrease, but Murphy's law* is always at play. Skateboarding, dieting and even **life is not about the falling off, it's about the very moment you hit the floor; it's what you do, how you react and your attitude that determine how your future is going to pan out**. My first stack was on Bondi Beach and shit, it hurt. My reaction? I laughed, I got back on and realized I probably should look out for potholes a bit more often. **Sometimes it's not a skill, but an attitude that develops us.**

My skateboard is checked in as an essential piece of kit for me when I travel. The underside has stickers from Los Angeles, Abu Dhabi and London. I'm very grateful to the version of me at twenty-seven who

---

* Murphy's law in essence is: whatever can go wrong, will go wrong.

kept getting up off the floor laughing, as without that attitude I would not enjoy my skates to the post office when the dreaded red slip of a missed parcel has been pushed through my letterbox.

Identification and Implementation

I do feel this wanting distraction more than development culture is something to worry about. YouTube, TikTok and Instagram provide constant hits of dopamine, while books, audiobooks, podcasts, courses and even picking up a new hobby like jiu jitsu could all provide just what your mind craves to realign your values, ethos and current beliefs. I feel we're bypassing the human psyche with social media, and although short term it could get you by, I don't think the long-term implications are healthy. It's a bit like having a meal-replacement shake: sure, for the odd meal it's OK, but if you remove all meals, your body may be getting what it 'technically' needs, but it's not how we evolved to eat.

I believe we are wired to get happiness from the simple pleasures in life. Watch how much kids enjoy a playfight or riding the dog like it's a horse. It makes me sad to see a baby with an iPad these days when they should be playing with Lego or eating grass because they saw the dog doing it (like I did as a child). I think that children should be building train tracks rather than tracking their finger across a screen on *Angry Birds*. I think that although we're adults, we need to identify that the same goes for us. Instead of a pint at the pub, where no doubt your phone will be sitting next to your beer glass, go for a sparring session with a friend. Or why not invite the same friend for a dog walk at a spot where you can see the sun go down. We can derive so much pleasure from a screen and grab that instant hit of dopamine, but for longevity I think we always prioritize the primal things that make us happy whenever the opportunity presents itself.

I'll talk about jiu jitsu again later in the book, but I never thought there would be a time in my life when I studied for a sport where small men (and some women) could beat me up, sit on me, choke me out and that I would call it the best sport I have ever played. Hobbies are not just distractions: they can be integral lessons in humility and respect.

When you're not out falling off your skateboard or scrolling social media, it's very important to take note of your mind and be present with what you're thinking. When you walk past a Ferrari you think: wow, nice car, and then move on with your day. However, when you scroll past a model on your Instagram feed in better shape than you, you take it personally, trying to suppress the feeling of jealousy, of feeling deflated, and from thereon in it amplifies. Before you know it, you're feeling flat from having seen the model you exposed yourself to, that you subscribed to and that you opted in to see. If we have the mental aptitude to walk past a nice car without letting it ruin our day, then **we must train our minds to do the same with what we subject ourselves to on social media**. It's imperative to stay above water within our culture of instant gratification, unobtainable goals and comparing ourselves to others to no avail.

Mindless assumptions

What is a mindless assumption? It's a subconscious thought that so many of us experience at one stage or another in our lives – an assumption and a standpoint that is inserted into the existing blueprint of life and one we need to challenge. It's things like the notion that we need an abundance of money, that we should aspire be famous, that we should aim to have our own property portfolio and retire without a mortgage, so we can travel and live the fullest life possible to the end of our days.

These views are my own. I only want to metaphorically shake the tree; if you remain clutching to the branch, that's cool and perhaps I'm incorrect. But if you feel like you're about to fall out of the tree, my job is done because I think you were clutching with a tight grip the wrong branch.

> *The last thing you should do in life is to climb to the very top of what you thought was the success ladder to find out you're at the top of the wrong ladder.*
>
> Paul Mort, friend and mentor

Mortgages

If you don't own a home at the point when you're reading this, I want to tell you that is fine, it's completely OK. For the longest part of human existence people didn't own their homes – it's a fairly recent thing, since the advent of credit. Credit is only a few hundred years old and it was the first time that humans traded money or resources without immediately being reimbursed by the other party.

I can't tell you what to buy or what not to; I can simply say where I stand on it and give you some ideas. Now, if you want to buy a Rolex or a sports car, it's absolutely your prerogative, but there's no stigma attached to being thirty-five and not having these things. People won't wonder, 'Where's their Rolex?' or, 'Where's their sports car?' However, with a mortgage, there's an invisible stigma, a feeling that you're not settled – even the idea that you could be unambitious, being mortgage-free at such a 'late stage' in life.

People will call their home their biggest investment, but equally it's their largest debt. Banks don't just lend money to people for the sake of spending money; for decades, they've loaned money to businesses so that the businesses can make money and repay them. But let's not overlook the fact that mortgages are one of the biggest money makers for banks. The American Dream of being a homeowner primarily benefits whoever sells you the mortgage in the first place. This isn't to say you can't make money on buying and selling a property, but it's important to point out that there are positives and negatives attached to this investment/large debt of 'owning' a home.

From a personality perspective, we're all very different, and some of us strive for security, while others don't. Some take a real sense of security in homeowning (and I'm not here to take that away from them), but others just don't feel obliged to make the commitment and I'm someone who sits in that category, not really caring that much about it. Renting a house is not 'throwing away money', as people say. It's having a place to live and to make memories in, somewhere to enjoy yourself and share space and time with someone you care about. For me, my twenties were amazing. I didn't save much money, I travelled a lot of the world, from surfing in Hawaii and playing rugby in New Zealand to going tubing in Laos (if you know, you know).

I could be wrong, but I just don't see many people really using that home investment to do anything with it. It's not like they'd sell up and travel or work through much of their bucket list. Often, people use their investment to upsize to a bigger house, maybe closer to a city that they work in. Home ownership is really part of a belief system; this is the point I want to make. Hundreds of thousands of pounds and all that really changes is the world's belief of who owns that home.

To me, whether I rent a property or own it when I'm in it, irrespective of the financial situation, the bed will still be as comfy, the shower as warm and the sofa as relaxing as it would be whatever the situation.

It's merely binary code in someone's server that changes because of the belief of ownership.

> The sum total of money in the world is about $60 trillion, yet the sum total of coins and banknotes is less than $6 trillion. More than 90 per cent of all money – more than $50 trillion appearing in our accounts – exists only on computer servers. Most business transactions are executed by moving electronic data from one computer file to another, without any exchange of physical cash.
>
> Yuval Noah Harari, *Sapiens: A Brief History of Humankind*

Maybe I am unique with my blasé approach to 'investment opportunities', but I think that's because I appreciate that 90 per cent of money isn't real – it doesn't exist. What is real to me is the sand between my toes on a beach, the moments at dinner with friends and the water as you jump into it from a boat. If you had the money to spare, sure, parking it in property is an option. But for most people, it isn't; they would need to make a substantial sacrifice in their younger and often responsibility-free years to put money aside to buy property, and I feel that does a lot of people a disservice. I don't own a property at the time of writing this book and I personally feel liberated by that, and I think if you're reading this and renting, you should, too. For sure, an investment opportunity has been missed, but rather that than a piece of life.

I'm not 'anti-mortgage'; I'm merely pro-choice and anti-stigma when it comes to property investment, especially for younger generations. In the blueprint for life that most follow, buying a property is far too high up on the list of things to do as a young adult, and I think other more important things should sit above it – enjoyment of work, travel, socializing and ensuring you don't wake up on any Mondays unhappy. If you experience wealth and can afford a house, great; if you inherit one, even better. But unfortunately, no one is guaranteed to live to the point when they will see off the biggest debt of their life. Should you kick it before setting up the appropriate paperwork, whoever you leave the property to will be stung with a 40 per cent inheritance tax (in the UK, anyway).

So, if you feel your personality traits suit security, absolutely seek a mortgage. If you feel like you desire freedom, there is nothing wrong with renting. And if your values align with not committing to a chunk of land and decades of debt, then do not feel bad about it. No number of properties can ensure happiness, fulfilment or a guarantee of the good life. So choose wisely and figure out what you want to do, not what others think you should do.

When I'm on my deathbed and my life flashes before my eyes, I very much doubt that owning a house will appear on that highlights reel.

Retirement

Growing old is a privilege denied to too many.

In essence, not everyone gets to grow old, we often forget that. None of us is safe from cancer, disease, a car crash or from being hit by the 191 bus that used to run down the road I grew up on as we're trying our new noise-cancelling headphones while crossing the road. I personally think about death fairly frequently because it helps me remain happy. Absurd? Not really – because if you think you're going to live for ever, like humans tend to do, you're already setting yourself up to fail.

If you think in this manner, whether you know it or not you are thinking you can do stuff 'someday' instead of now.

For all of the most important things, the timing always sucks. Waiting for a good time to quit your job? The stars will never align and the traffic lights of life will never all be green at the same time. The universe doesn't conspire against you, but it doesn't go out of its way to line up the pins either.

Conditions are never perfect. 'Someday' is a disease that will take your dreams to the grave with you. Pro and con lists are just as bad. If it's important to you and you want to do it 'eventually', just do it and correct the course along the way.

Timothy Ferriss, *The 4-Hour Work Week*

Knowing you're going to either be old sooner than you think or dead sooner than you ever imagined is actually a great incentive to get shit done right now. As I mentioned earlier, Parkinson's law states that tasks take up whatever time we allocate to them to complete. Similar to only having an hour to get work done and the productivity that comes with that, we should not be ignorant of the fact that we may not have as much time as we think. I often think to myself: I'll construct the perfect life up until fifty and anything beyond that is a bonus.

Before you think that Elon Musk is going to come up with an eco-friendly invention that enables us to live for ever, think this: if you live to be the oldest out of all your friends and family, you'll get to see them all die, which is probably worse than the thought of dying itself.

I truly believe that what makes things beautiful is the notion that we may not get to see or do that thing again. Let's imagine you quit the job you hate, you take your former mortgage savings and fly to Bali to stay in a hostel. Then on your last night in Bali, you drink a Bintang beer at the beach on a bean bag with the stray dog you made friends with. You take a deep breath and, as you finish the beer and turn your back on the beach, you have this feeling deep inside, as you take one little glance over your shoulder, that there's every chance you may not make it back and see it all again. That, in itself, is what makes the moment magical; the false notion that you're going to see it again for sure can ruin the moment. I have that feeling every time I watch a sunset in Bali. And I'll never forget the moment either, because it's one that makes me happy, knowing how lucky I am to make it to that beach* in the first place.

I know there are people at home saving for a mortgage and they probably won't ever go to Bali, as it's a 'bit far away for a holiday', especially since they only have five days of annual leave left to play with. You see, they probably went to their mate's wedding a few months ago (who has since got divorced) and used up a lot of their holiday on that. Not to mention that they probably had their hand forced by their employer to take the days off between Christmas and New Year, so the office could remain closed. It's those people I want to wake up in this part of the book. So many people go to the same boring place year on year because it's easy – not just easy to travel, but easy to take their minds off their existing lives, which, quite frankly, they're bored of.

The average retirement age in the United Kingdom is 64.5 years old. Why? Because at that age people are nearing a fifty-year tenure of working each fucking day for money. My question is this: why do we wait so long to do what we want to do in retirement?

What is on most people's retirement lists? I asked my followers on social media and they said: travel, adventure, sleep, live in France, play

---

* Since writing this, the very beach I named 'dog beach' no longer exists and some fancy hotels have been built on it. I will forever cherish the last moment I spent on those bean bags with the dog. Like I said, as I left, the thought of maybe never seeing it again (nor the dog) was what made it so special.

golf, spend time with friends, live on a farm … But the best answer I got was this: 'hopefully everything will be done at that point'.

If I let you in on a little secret it's this: avoid the five-star resorts in Bali – that's not where the magic is. It's the bean bags, the wooden shacks and the backpackers, when you are with twenty strangers from all across the world, and you're all a little unsure about what you're doing in life, but that is what makes you somehow vulnerable and all weirdly connected. There is no age restriction on an adventure, there is no prejudice when travelling, and when you're in these hostels, you all share similar vulnerabilities and it brings you together. My last stint in a hostel was at the age of twenty-seven – there were people ten years my junior in the same dorm and no one cared.

During COVID-19, there was a weird sensation of the world being slightly peaceful because we all shared the exact same problem for once, a problem not broken up by borders, language, race or political standpoints. And you find the same thing when you travel solo as a backpacker at any age: you all share the same itch, the same desire, the same hunger for that beer on a beanbag, and you feel suffocated by the notion of a thirty-to-forty-year stint before you can see what you want to see right now. You sit there, you look around and you wonder: why are the other members of the herd not sharing this suffocated feeling? You think that those deserted beaches won't be deserted for ever; last year's paradise is already a party island. And social media means there are no longer 'secret' destinations to discover. Waiting cannot be an option. Why is everyone waiting to be sixty-five to do this?

When I am sixty-five it will be 2054. The population is estimated to grow to 9.9 billion by that point. Just looking at all that happened in 2020 alone, you can see why I don't trust the future enough to hedge my bets on waiting that long. It makes no sense.

When you hit thirty, you realize two things: firstly, it's only going to get harder – waking up, peeing in the middle of the night and the random lower-back pain from, well … life itself. The second thing is thinking: fuck, I'm not even halfway to retirement yet (even less when you account for just your professional life).

I can't imagine many sixty-five-year-olds learning to ride a moped for the first time or going skinny dipping with a group of people they just met. I see the travellers sitting on the floor at the airport, and I see how 'normal' members of society look at them, like they're lost in life.

I watch them look and I smile to myself – because I was once in silk trousers on the floor of Bangkok Airport. I've lived both lives first-hand and let me tell you this: it's often the guys travelling in suits who are the lost ones in life; they probably have a mortgage and an overpriced suit skewing their perception of what true success, wealth and happiness really are – a bit like a magnet next to a compass. Find me a miserable backpacker; I'll wait.

Again, I'm not attacking you if you haven't travelled. I'm just pointing out that in life this blueprint lets too many people down. We're made to feel like we're missing something if we don't have the dream family where everyone gets on and has pancakes together for breakfast. We're made to feel like we should own the home and have the nine-to-five job. But remember what Bill Burr said about sleeping on a futon when you're thirty (see page 46).

My dad is now retired. He spent fifty years working in the same job, and I will admit that he really is happy to be retired. However, he also loved every moment in his job and took complete satisfaction from it. But he has never used social media, and I feel he and his generation are potentially the last who can actually retire properly and be happy with it. Because the younger generations today are faster-paced, dopamine hitting and social-media driven, and I just don't think the model of work

160

and retirement is going to suit the psyche of the modern-day millennial. I think it's foolish to put all the eggs in the basket of later life – it's a gamble at best, and one slip-up in your forties and you may not be able to climb Machu Picchu with that dodgy hip that gets sore climbing stairs.

For most of my dad's career he'd fly to countries all around the world just to meet people. But now we have the Internet, we have Zoom meetings and the capability for so many professions to work remotely. I don't see why more businesses aren't letting their workforces work from abroad. Working for fifty years and then having the rest of the time off is a bit too extreme for me. Again, going on holiday can bore a lot of people, as they go from too much work to not enough. I wish we could trial a new model whereby travel could be permitted for the workforce as long as they got the work done. Imagine how that would benefit the mental health and productivity of workforces around the world. For professions where that's not possible we should be giving people more holiday each year. Better yet, let's give people/employees more autonomy over their holidays and free time. Some businesses are now trialling this and letting their workforce have more control over their own time, but in most cases it still remains the opposite. So many workforces prioritize call stats over work–life balance.

You think I'm mad, don't you? *That's ridiculous, James, that's absurd. It's OK for you, James,* etc. But I say this because the existing model is not working for us. The reason I don't want people to wait until they're older is because there is a fundamental fault in that, I am afraid.

The leading cause of death in the United Kingdom between the ages of 20 and 34 is suicide; in Australia it's the leading cause of death for adults between 15 and 44. (See References, p. 256.)

Do you see how I may draw the conclusion that saving it all for the end may not be the best decision for your time on Earth as a human being? Now, again, I may be wrong, but I just want some of you to wake up to the fact that you really do need to control your work life as best you can. If there is any opportunity to work remotely, try to negotiate even a day at home a week, ensure you're extra productive on that day and build the case to work from home as much as possible. (And choose a plain backdrop for your Zoom calls, so that your boss doesn't clock the fact that you're in Greece or Spain on a Thursday.)

Of course, there are a lot of workers who can't work remotely, such as people who work in the police or nurses and doctors (and I'm grateful they're not prescribing me antibiotics from the other side of the world). But there are so many people who need to realize we don't live to work – we work to live.

Think of anyone you have ever met. Is there anyone who regrets taking some time to travel when they're younger rather than older? Ask them. And I know you're thinking: not everyone can just up and leave, James. Well, I get that. But if you work your arse off for a few years, options will appear – if you're that good at your job, they'll do anything to keep you, even letting you work remotely for a few months every year. And if there's currently no scope in your line of work to do so, find a way. I feel like if I put a gun to your head to make you do it, you'd find one.

I see a lot of people experience anxiety with their work, their future and their direction. Worrying about whether to pursue a potentially better job, something that's a closer fit and more aligned with what they want to do. They'll say, 'I really love my job. I've been there several years, and I get on with everyone really well. I don't know what to do!' I'll say to them, 'Well … go for the new job! Because if it turns out to be a mistake, you can pursue other opportunities; you'll actually have to take risks, put yourself out there and go for it.' Professional lives do not favour those who stay in the same place for ever. It's an important part of life to change your surroundings. Also, it's worth noting that there is no longer such a stigma attached to having several job changes on your CV. For instance, if you sat in an interview and someone asked you why you only lasted a month in your previous or current role, you could say, 'Well, I expected the job to be like this … however, I didn't feel it was right for me and I'm not the type of person to work a job I am not passionate about. So, I am here to see if I can bring my passion to the opportunity you have available.' You cannot be faulted for that. The last type of person anyone wants to hire is one who'd sit in a job they disliked for several years on end, worried more about how their CV looks.

Any person's value within an organization is determined by how hard they work and their attitude. Whether you're in your first job behind a bar, stacking shelves in a supermarket or washing cars, do the best fucking job you can. It's important, because for a lot of you that attitude will transfer into your next job, then the one after that. The focus of your mind should be on this, not retirement; it should be about tomorrow and turning up with your head screwed on. I worked in a bar for years, and I would take pride in pouring a bloody good pint. It wasn't what I wanted to do in life, but I kept the bar clean, wiped surfaces when I wasn't asked to and ensured I remembered people's orders to make them feel that bit more at home in the pub. My mind never drifted to my sixties; it remained in the present, in the attitude of doing a good job each day.

Waiting for retirement to me seems like a lifestyle trap that only benefits employers in big companies and, of course, those who benefit from taxation of pension pots. You can keep your idealism of retirement if you would like to, but I'll work until my final days. Work is about taking daily satisfaction in doing the best job possible each and every day. And I believe it's a little bit sad to think about a life without that. I think that's how the human brain works, too – instead of just crossing a finishing line at the end of a marathon absolutely shattered, we should keep going; it doesn't have to be at the same pace, but I certainly don't think we aim for a void in life with no purpose at the end. So instead of sprinting only to land flat on your face at the finish line, why not slow the race down, take it gently, enjoy every mile, stop and smile at things along the way. With that attitude, you'll more than likely want to continue the journey beyond that final ribbon.

Success, Conversions and Satisfaction

'Will you follow me, James?'

Sandra, 37, from Norwich

That is a classic example of the new era of narcissistic quantification of self-worth, based on an arbitrary number of people who opt in to see your posts. We have this false idealism that we need loads of these to be successful, and people share this idealism **even if they don't work online**.

We, then, are in the midst of the selfie era. I love every selfie I have with someone – to this day, it's still a mix of weird and wonderful at the same time. There are theories on why people want them and the association of lifting your own status, but to me, I think it's an entry-level way for people to just have the confidence to say hello.

It's mad. People get really upset if you unfollow them, too. Let's be honest, being followed in real life is something you'd never want, yet someone you went to school with doesn't want to see pictures of your cat and you take it to heart. It's each person's prerogative what they want to see in their social-media feed – they may be seeking daily inspiration, fitness ideas or even just a distraction from their own lifestyle, and no matter how wonderful your cat is, they may not want to see it.

There are certain apps on smartphones that actually notify you when someone unfollows you. Now, this is a prime example of opening the door to unhappiness. Is there any scenario where an unfollow would make you happy? No. Therefore, every unfollow makes you unhappy. You went out of your way to download an app that makes you unhappy, well done. And there are several websites purely for people to gossip about people anonymously, too. They are hotspots for trolls. Yet you'll find people's egos get the better of them and they'll proactively seek out someone's negative opinion of them. And rarely does anyone walk away without damaged self-esteem.

Around once a year, I run a 'B2B' (business to business) event for personal trainers where I help them develop their companies. I need people to operate well, so they don't go out of business. If they continue to do as they do currently, it leaves the fitness industry with a huge churn rate that serves no one well. Not only that, but you can be in incredible shape but not know your arse from your elbow when it comes to how to operate a good strategy in business. One of the craziest things to this day is how much personal trainers worry about what other personal trainers think of their work, when **funnily enough they are the only people who will never do business with them**. Worrying over the only people who won't pay them – exhausting, right? I love these opportunities to realign their mindset with what's important and move them away from what isn't – very similar to what I am doing here with you.

I'm so surprised about how often people ask me, 'James, how do I get more followers?' The number of times I have had well-established and recognized coaches say this, too. I ask them how many they currently have and they'll say 5,000, for example; but they see the popular coaches of the world with much higher followings and think they do not have enough, that their following count is inadequate and insufficient for success. This is incorrect. I tell these coaches, 'Hold on, if you converted 1 per cent of your following – just 1 per cent – you'd need to hire someone.' It's never a follower problem, it's a conversion problem.*

So, let's say from an online perspective that person had 1 per cent of their social-media following doing 'business' with them. As an online coach, I charged £65 (118 AU$) a week, the same as I charged for one hour of my time, and I promised they'd have that on a weekly basis. For this person to do business with his following, that's £3,250 (5,910 AU$) a week, £169,000 (307,350 AU$) a year. But let's be honest, who wants to work fifty hours a week? £84,500 (153,675 AU$) would be a much better figure for half the hours, twenty-five each week, which is five a day, AND you could do that completely online, taking the weekends off. Telling me you need more followers? You're kidding me, mate.

Tell you what, while we're here, let's open this conversation up further: how about £42,250 (76,837 AU$) for two and a half hours' work a day?

Now, if I asked you which salary you'd want, you'd automatically pick the biggest, right? But who is truly richest in the three scenarios if I took the finances away? Sure, Mr £160,000 gets to stay in the nicest hotel and drive the most expensive car, whereas Mr £40,000 may stay somewhere a little cheaper but has the majority of his day to travel, walk, read, listen to and do whatever he pleases. Wealth and financial status are vastly different in my eyes.

So, I rarely find people who need more followers. They may need to market themselves better, work on converting their existing following to paying customers, but that's marketing, not just following. I know

---

* As mentioned previously, it's perspective here that's the issue: comparing their following to someone else's, taking it to heart and using it as a reason why they're not doing well right now. You don't need a big following to do well in business; it helps, but it's not essential.

what you're thinking. Where did I learn about marketing myself to where I am now? Well, I decided to be Mr £40,000 for a while and absorbed books and podcasts when I was working only two to five hours a day, travelling in Bali and Australia. As I have said, your trajectory is far more important than where you currently are; you can always make more money, but you can't always have more time.

TASK

You can do this whether you are self-employed or work for an organization – try answering by adapting the goals to apply to your ambitions. What if I told you that there are three ways to grow a business?

1. Get your clients to buy more from you (new product offering).
2. Get your clients to buy more frequently from you.
3. Get new clients.

Two-thirds of your business exists within your current client base, yet what do most businesses seek? New clients and more followers. See where not only time can be wasted here, but also valuable energy? The most important thing for me wasn't the business side but the client side. Having a smaller group of people who I would give more time and attention to was crucial. In a service-based industry like personal training, you only really need ten clients to succeed. If I had ten clients seeing me for three sessions a week, that is. If I served those with a multifaceted approach to solve as many problems as possible, I would not only be preserving my own energy but at the same time giving a better service,

---

which means those ten clients could achieve the best success. I do see a lot of people trying to spread themselves very thin and that's always going to be a lot harder. Whether you're a painter/decorator, IT sales executive or a dog walker, valuing your existing client base will always trump your endless efforts to find new ones.

'Wealth' 2.0

As we have seen, the one with the most money is not always the richest. Remember the situation regarding how many online clients a person could have? Work–life balance can't be quantified by your bank balance. I am afraid more isn't always better. When you hear how much someone earns you're not often also told about the headaches, stress or sacrifices that may have been made for that wealth.

A very strange phenomenon is that whether you earn £5,000 (9,000 AU$) a month or £25,000, life doesn't change that much. You see more go to the tax man, but life remains very similar. Ask ten people what they'd ask a genie in a lamp for and I bet nine would say they want to be millionaires without a thought.

Why are we fixated on an amount of money which wouldn't actually change our lives that much? The hardest part for me is that people don't actually want the money; they want the life that they think someone who has that amount of money has. Getting paid a big or small salary must be seen in the context of how much you like your work. Getting paid £25k a year for something you love is much better than being paid £100k a year for something you hate; you may just have a less expensive watch and you'll probably stay in a less glamorous hotel on holiday, but ultimately, your watch will still tell the time and the hotel will still provide a good night's sleep.

I always advise people to have work that they're passionate about, so it doesn't feel like work. As the saying goes, 'Work a job you love and you'll never work a day in your life.' If you are going to work in a profession that brings you no passion, the solution is not to spend too much time doing it. It's a bit like exercise – a lot of people don't enjoy it, but as long as they can get it done in a short period of time they learn to love it because they can get on with their lives outside of it. If you're in a profession that takes up a lot of time but generates very little passion, you're ultimately selling your time for money and that, in my opinion, is not a good way to do it.

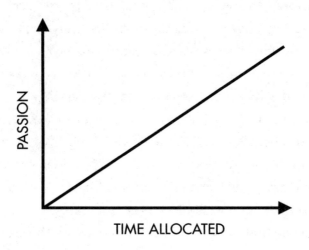

A hugely sobering podcast for me was when a friend, mentor and peer named Paul Mort did a podcast about his business turning over its first million. His question was not about what to spend it on but instead: 'Was it all worth it?' And after a silence, he said, 'I'm not sure, you know.' He spoke about the number of times he'd snapped at his kids for wanting his attention and all the times he hadn't been the best husband or father. And for what? Money? Arguably, he was a man primarily looking to support his family, yet neglecting them in a bid to do so.

Guess what else they never tell you? However much money you earn, you'll get used to it very fast. It's known as regression to the mean.

If you buy a Ferrari, you will get bored of it; if you downsize, you will get used to it; if you lose a limb or win the lottery, in six months it will feel normal. It is a part of being human. And whatever financial figure you set your sights on, you will get used to it. I always remind myself when I look at world-class models that there's someone out there bored of fucking them. Harsh but true.

On the flip side, we have adaptability. Earlier, we talked about the frog which doesn't notice if you heat the water around it slowly. Well, some people adapt to jobs that make them miserable; there's an arbitrary pay rise or a bigger cubicle and before long it's become the norm. They think that's just what their job is. We see this in relationships, too, where you ask yourself, 'If it was like this when I first met them, would I still be involved?'

We're very fickle by nature and we succumb to another cognitive bias known as the 'hot-cold empathy gap'. **When we're hot, it's hard to imagine being cold, when we're tired, it's hard to think about being energized and vice versa.** When we're hard up financially, we can't imagine what it's like to have disposable income and it becomes a dream state which the lottery ticket could buy a way into. However, let's say we win the lottery, we'll very soon forget what it was like to be hard up and the magical sensation will evaporate.

It's human nature, so before you opt for the next highest-paying job that may not give you any intrinsic happiness or much of a work–life balance, please keep it in mind. The only thing you won't get bored of is a job that doesn't feel like work, whether that's done from your laptop, hustling online or in a dog rescue kennel. Whatever it is, you wear the ultimate wealth not on your wrist, but on your face, in the form of a smile – because ultimate wealth is having a life you love. Being a millionaire doesn't save you from depression; it's not the money you need at the end of the day, just a different perception on what to prioritize for yourself and yourself only in this journey we all know and share as life.

The pleasure black hole

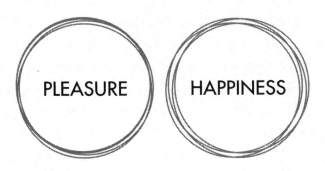

One important thing to realize is that there is a difference between pleasure and happiness. It's about instant versus long-term gratification – understanding that happiness is a perspective, an attitude and can be accomplished with a certain mindset. When you have that perspective, you can go after real wealth, and it's better than simply just being rich.

Pleasure can be nights out, expensive things, designer clothes and holidays. By no means is this a bad thing – I mean if you ever buy something from Gucci, the effort that goes into the wrapping alone is sometimes worth the cost! But you don't *need* pleasure. Sure, it helps, but you need to remain aware that it's a black hole* that consumes all in its path.

---

* The gravitational pull of a black hole is so vast not even light can escape (hence the black appearance); you can't see it, you can only feel its presence.

And as a black hole would increase in mass through absorbing whatever comes its way, it would, in theory, then develop a stronger gravitational pull over time. This is not intended to put you off the pursuit of pleasure, just to give you an understanding of how I view it. **You can elicit satiety in many areas of life, but pleasure is one to be aware and wary of.** If you seek happiness from pleasure with gambling, drug use and partying, you may lose sight of what really makes you happy and end up depressed, hungover and broke because of it.

> The largest black holes are called 'supermassive'. These black holes have masses that are more than 1 million suns together. Scientists have found proof that every large galaxy contains a supermassive black hole at its centre. The supermassive black hole at the centre of the Milky Way galaxy is called Sagittarius A. It has a mass equal to about 4 million suns. [See References, p. 256.]

I think as long as people have the right perception of pleasure, they can make better and more rational decisions. Take gambling, for example. I rarely gamble, but before I do, I think to myself: James, this is not ultimately going to make you happy, but it may bring you twenty minutes of pleasure. What is that worth? £10, cool. Be prepared to lose it, and if you walk away with nothing, you bought yourself a short stint of pleasure.

A night out? Pleasure. Getting a bit drunk? Pleasure. Holidays in a really expensive hotel? Pleasure. I'm well aware that the money that's in my pocket or that's paying for the poolside bar tab is going into a black hole and won't make its way back any time soon, but it weirdly makes me feel better about spending it that way, too.

Raising a family? Now that's not pleasure. That's happiness (for most people, anyway).

Happiness is also sitting on the beach with one of your best friends, thinking the shit out of life because the life you have constructed permits you to do so. Happiness is a state of mind, not an occasion. It's wanting what you already have, it's gratitude on a constant basis. We go through life finding what makes us happy and also finding what doesn't; sometimes that takes years, as we'll see in the next chapter.

Fucking

This is a topic that has been discussed recently in terms of toxic masculinity, and I think it's important to consider it within this framework – to look at how society and culture create unhealthy mindsets for adolescents and young adults. For many years, like many other guys, I just loved getting laid. I felt accomplished every time it happened. I had made it a value for success, through following the herd and what my friends were doing. You got laid, you got a high five the next morning with the lads. I remember keeping a rough tally of how many women I'd slept with in my late teens, and I'll never forget the moment (some years on) when I hit what I believed to be 100.

I was in my mid-twenties when the 'century' happened. I had supposedly conquered what so many men hadn't and wouldn't. I remember seeing a statistic that the average man slept with just seven women and I thought to myself how well I'd done to beat that average by ninety-three. I recognize my finite mindset and way of thinking now. I was treating it like a game that could be won – which it can't.

Do you want to know what happens when you reach your century? **Absolutely fucking nothing.** No one is there at the finish line, no one is clapping, no one is high fiving you with a smile on their face. You can't cash in your 'lad points' – and you realize that you've accomplished absolutely nothing. What I thought was winning was not; what I thought was a successful stint turned out to be a hollow and empty realization. I had climbed a ladder in life to get to the top, only to find that I didn't want to be there. I'd created a game in my head no one else was playing – no one was winning, no one was losing – and I'd done it all in a bid to feed my own ego and not my ambitions. I was playing 'the invisible game' (see p. 107), but with the wrong value in mind.

I came to realize that I had been chasing a very poor value, based on what I believed everyone else had also been basing their values on. I had a long, hard think to myself about the value – where had it come from? Why was it ingrained in me as a youngster? And why had no one taken the opportunity to remove it from my mind? Why hadn't someone somewhere stopped me to say, 'James, no one cares about this apart from you and your ego. This will not make you any happier.'

It was a value that I came to discover only sets people up for what I believe to be an unhappy life. I don't know anyone truly happy on their own growing old and using regular 'one nighters' of meaningless sex as a constituent of the good life. They pretend it is, they allow their friends to live vicariously through their antics, but deep down they probably are waiting for the 'right partner' when what they need is the 'right values'.

In truth, the ones who have the young family and the partners – they are the true winners. I know married people can very rarely have sex, especially with a young family, but at least their encounter has some fucking meaning to it, some passion and you'd hope some love. A lot of marriages end up in divorce, and that's OK, too. At least there was something that was magical at some point, and if there are kids, they have something to share and a joint interest in bringing up those small people together. I don't think anyone truly envies someone whose only accomplishments are how often they get laid, though.

Ultimately, I learned that the only thing I'd truly accomplished was a very awkward conversation that I'm going to have with my future wife. I do hope she can just see past the fact that I was unaware of what a poor value for success sex was, and that she should, if anything, be happy that I see past that now. So, my future wife, if you're reading this …

… You're welcome. It's out my system. There, you can see the classic way you can turn any negative into a positive with the right angle. So many of the things we hate we can, in fact, be very grateful for. So, remember, if your partner has had a lot of sexual encounters, it's not a fault in them, but probably a fault in their values. (I'll get on to this a little later in the book in more detail.)

Fucking people should be a part of the process to find the person who is ultimately right for you. If it feels right, go for it – don't be fixed and afraid to fail. And if it all ends in tears, just remember you're learning who's not right for you, and we like learning, because learning ultimately makes us happy, right?

Don't worry about the past of someone you like, and the few or many encounters that have led them to be there with you and not someone else each night. Insecurities are human nature, but park them alongside the old values you may have held close, as they will not bring you any closer to a happy life.

Finally, on fucking, there's no point working your whole life to accomplish so much and do great things, only to experience those things alone, is there? Human beings are sociable creatures and the perfect partner gives you someone to share those great times with. The 'lad' culture might work for your twenties and, I suppose, your early thirties, but eventually, the hard-man façade needs to be parked by us men, and we need to realize that women run the world – they're just smart enough to let us men think we're in charge.

PART V

COMFORT ZONES AND ESCAPISM

In this chapter, I'm going to bring science into the fray to get you to stop attaching so much significance to things that don't deserve it. An informative science lesson awaits with important points to be taken away from it.

A Brief Introduction to Physics (and Getting to Know Your Comfort Zone)

I need you to understand that some things exist and some things don't. We have matter and non-matter, which is a simple classification. The table I sit my laptop on as I write this is matter. It exists, people can see it and anyone can touch it. Your car is made out of matter, as are you.

Anything that takes up space and has mass is matter.

Now, there are also things that are non-matter. For instance, time, sound, sunlight, reflection, gravity, memories, dreams, love and heat. We cannot touch them; some can be felt, but do not exist outside of our perception of simple atoms.

I've touched briefly on a sense of finitism* and the mindset with which many people approach their lives, thinking they can win things they can't and that they can come out on top of things that physically can't be won, like social media or relationships.

A comfort zone is not derived of matter. Yet we often act like it is. There are laws of nature and physics that govern our universe and we seem to think that our limiting beliefs and fabricated comfort zones

---

* Rejection of the belief that anything can actually be infinite.

wield the same power and limitations as these. But they do not. Unless we allow them to. The speed of light* is set, and we cannot travel at that speed, ever. That's not down to technological advancements, either. For many years, I was gutted that I never flew on a Concorde plane. When it was removed from circulation in 2003, I felt like we had really taken a backward step. For the first time ever, we got slower. In my mind, I have always thought it's just a waiting game, and soon enough we will have the technological advancement to travel at the speed of light.

It's not technology, though. It's a law of physics. You see, as I just touched on, things that contain matter – such as us and the spaceship we'd have in space – consist of matter and would also have mass. Without getting into a physics class, imagine this: as objects travel faster and faster, they get heavier and heavier – the heavier they get, the harder it is to achieve acceleration. So, you never get to the speed of light because the mass of the object becomes too much. Light does not contain mass as it's non-matter. Therefore, sadly, I'm here to tell you that we cannot ever travel anywhere near the speed of light.

I'll get to my point shortly, but I do love space, so I must share with you one more interesting fact to bring up next time you end up lying on the grass, looking at the stars, chatting waffle about space. So, hypothetically speaking – and only hypothetically speaking – if we could travel at the speed of light, it would take six months to accelerate to that speed, and even then, that's if we accelerate at 1g-force (which is constant acceleration relative to what we would experience as gravity at the back of the spaceship). So, even if we had the technology to

---

* The speed of light is 299,792.458 kilometres per second. Before the 1600s most people assumed light moved instantaneously. Galileo was among the first to think that light travelled at a finite speed, finitism at its finest.

accelerate that fast, it would take a year – six months of constant accel-eration, followed by six months of constant deceleration. If we were to travel at twice that speed, sure, we could get it all done in three months each way, but you'd spend half a year weighing twice your bodyweight (2g-force), not ideal in the slightest, even in space. OK, I'll get to my point now.

There are laws in place within our universe that stop us from doing things, but outside of that? Well, everything is possible. **Now, what I want to ask you is this: where is your comfort zone?**

Think about it. It does not exist. It is non-matter, like time, created by us and relative to us. However, time helps us; comfort zones do not. **You cannot touch your comfort zone, yet I bet you let it act upon you like a physical law of the universe far stronger than gravity.** In your head you give it the same power as any of Newton's laws. I want you to really understand this: the barriers we are holding up do not exist, but they are so ingrained inside us that it can feel like they are a part of our DNA. It's important that we challenge the notion of our actual boundaries. Again, if we took them to court, I am sure we'd be laughed out of there with no evidence to prove why we can't do things when we put our minds to it (bar travelling faster than light, that is).

We remain in our zones of comfort because we believe they will keep us safe. The very same instinct that says no to a bungee jump or turns down the offer of a sky dive. But it's not just life-threatening actions that our minds reject; it is just about anything that could make us feel uncomfortable or any scenario in which we may not succeed. It's an instinctual and primitive drive to be risk averse.

For instance, a risk-averse investor might choose to put their money into a bank account with a low but guaranteed interest rate rather than into a stock that has high expected returns but a higher chance of potentially losing value. Human beings are risk averse by nature. This can be seen in the sport of Brazilian jiu jitsu, too. Any offensive move comes with a risk – the more offensive, the greater the risk; so, you have to learn your way out of sticky situations and you can play your opponent on him being risk-averse with a lot of his passes, submissions or takedowns. We fear losing things more than we value gaining something of the same worth; knowing how the human mind deals with risk is one of the best places to attempt to submit someone in the sport – just as they're losing their grip on something they have worked hard for they will more often than not make an irrational decision because of it. I'll talk about jiu jitsu again a bit later, but for now, I want you to realize that being risk averse is in your DNA; you're not broken – it's just something we all succumb to naturally.

Imagine this for a second: you have a strong opinion on something that you want to share with more people. Whether it's a blog, a vlog, a tweet, you will, of course, be crippled by the fear of someone disagreeing. But the urge to share isn't based on the person who disagrees; it's about airing your view to see if someone else feels the same, to know you're not alone. And it could liberate that stranger to know that *they're* not alone with *their* opinion either, potentially bringing the two of you together. What is there to lose in this scenario? Someone disagreeing with you is not a loss; it's not a slur on your identity. I am sure Marmite do not lose sleep over all the people who do not like the taste of it, as there are so many who do.

Social media can float trolls from the deepest corners of the Internet, but that shouldn't kill your urge to share your opinion. Your views could help someone, make them smile, realign their train of thought – yet so many tweets, podcasts and blogs are never sent, recorded or posted because our comfort zones hold us back.

Blogging, posting, airing your opinions strengthens your identity over time, as you become able to do these things less fearfully with each one. The worst-case scenario is never that bad and bolstering your identity in this way will only build who you are as a person. And after doing it repeatedly, you'll probably feel more inclined to try other things that are usually outside of your (fabricated) comfort zone, such as asking for a pay rise or a promotion or for a phone number.

You may decide you want to record your first ever video for social media, to promote your business selling massage balls, spare motorcycle parts or even legal services, for example. You want to use the video to help people get to know who you are, but you're scared and rightly so. They don't teach you how to talk to camera, and I certainly had to learn for myself. As you hit record, you stutter, lose the ability to speak or get your thoughts in order. Your worst-case scenario is that your first video isn't that polished and not many people see it – and that's not the end of the world because even armed with three views you just got better at speaking to the camera. What a worst-case scenario that is.

What if I told you there is no boundary, nothing you can't do, nothing that will make you uncomfortable unless you let it? What if I said that to become comfortable with doing uncomfortable things all you have to do is get familiar with them through repetition?

If you try and you fail, the repercussions are rarely negative, and most likely your situation will be improved. Nothing is stopping you from speaking in front of a crowd, maintaining eye contact with a stranger or giving someone your number. If there was a law of science dictating the rules of what comfort zones are, I'm sure scientists would have found out about it by now, aren't you?

Escapism

Escapism is mental diversion from unpleasant or boring aspects of daily life, typically through activities involving imagination or entertainment.

Let's look at online gaming for a start. There have been numerous studies on the addictive qualities of online gaming and their psychosocial effect on users, but I think we'll just call a spade a spade and see it as a form of escapism. Without context, it's impossible to say whether or not gaming would benefit or damage someone's learning, development or social skills, but every human being should be allowed to have their own form of escapism as their prerogative. For some this could be fishing, for others gaming or yoga or meditation.

I think it's important that we empathize before judging someone's method of escapism and try to understand why they are doing it. I've been guilty before of prioritizing video gaming over quality time with a loved one; that doesn't mean I love playing *Call of Duty* more than I care about the loved one, but it's a nice way for me to switch off from whatever else I am doing in the 'normal' world. **We're all uniquely different, so we must try to understand that when someone just wants to disconnect from the day-to-day – say, with a glass of wine and a book – it's not something to be taken personally; it's just a form of escapism, and we all need that at times.** I've noted that a lot of athletes I know play video games, too. It makes sense because of how athletes are wired mentally, always wanting to win and be the best. If your coach says you need to go rest, you may need something to shift your focus for the rest of the afternoon, and as your body repairs, you may seek your wins elsewhere, online.

Other forms of escapism can be sexually orientated, with role play, for instance. However, I'm not so well versed on that, so I'll leave it for someone else's book. Something I have experienced first-hand, though, is the escapism associated with drinking. We often so easily intertwine alcohol with social life, then social life with 'culture'.

We say it is sociable and we use it on social occasions, but when you really think about it, it's anti-social.

I drink. I love to drink occasionally, but do you know what drunk people are when you're sober? Annoying. However, we drink and label it 'social' because it allows us to dull emotions and, even better, to break down our own comfort zones. For example, we often associate it with giving us the courage to talk to someone we wouldn't usually approach. With alcohol, we become audacious, willing and brave. Beer goggles often help the situation, too. When we do it enough and see it around us, it's then intertwined as part of our culture. But really it's just a joint collective of people trying to escape to another reality where they can accomplish more outside of their comfort zones.

Some people turn to alcohol to escape a reality which many tell themselves they want to be in when they don't. I think people really need to realize that sometimes they can be drinking for the wrong reasons. To escape a zone that doesn't physically exist? That's not a good deal. To escape a life that doesn't stimulate you? That's also not a good deal.

Want to know something that rocked me when I hit thirty? A simple sentence that really changed a lot of things: **would I enjoy this sober?** If it's a nice dinner with friends and another bottle of wine is being ordered, I think to myself: absolutely. If it's walking into a club three hours later than when I'd usually be going to sleep, I think it'd be an absolute nightmare.

Recreational drug use often occurs when people are trying to escape from a situation in their lives. This needs to be identified because, ultimately, some wounds need more than to be covered with a plaster. It's often the easy solution, but sometimes you need to identify if something is more severe and therefore needs stitches, for instance. No one wants stitches, but if you want the wound to heal properly, you need to do more than just cover it up with a plaster and hoping for the best.

Priorities

What we prioritize is hugely important, obviously. But I feel like many people are prioritizing the wrong things in life.

Let's delve into work as an example. The first figure you look at is how much you'd get paid a year for the job. There's no quantification of the stress associated with it, how much time it will occupy your brain out of hours, not even an enjoyment factor. Just responsibilities, role and on-target earnings (OTE). When we search for a job, we set the income as a priority in most cases, and we think of linear earning increases and 'opportunities'. Are these good priorities? Are there more important things to put first? Like a commute? Enjoyability? Passion for the organization?

Corporate work is a relatively new thing to humans, and we don't appreciate that enough. For most of our existence we worked in tribes, gathering food, making fires and surviving. We didn't clock in and out of foraging or get into trouble for sleeping in. I think when it comes to prioritizing our professional lives there are more important things than salary. Those who get paid the most don't always enjoy their work the most – an almost sobering reality, isn't it?

Now, let's ask ourselves why is it that we prioritize anything ahead of our mental health?

In the event of a plane crash you're told to put the oxygen mask on yourself first before helping others, the reason being that if you lose consciousness you can't help anyone around you. This logic should be carried over to our mental health and daily lives – because our mental health is the cornerstone of our wellbeing. There is no financial sum, trip to Vegas or any other materialistic item that can save you from suffering with poor mental health. That's not to say it's just about priorities, but they have a big part to play. The universe is 14 billion years old, and you'll get 100 of those if you're incredibly lucky. The human brain can't quite compute billions of years; I always remember Neil deGrasse Tyson explaining it this way (see References, p. 256):

> If an American football field were a timeline of the 14-billion-year-old Universe, with the Big Bang at one end, then at the other end, the width of a single blade of grass spans 30,000 years of human history, from the earliest humans to the present.

So, when we look at how long we're alive for, it's the tiniest fraction (0.0000007142 per cent) of the existence of the universe so far. I think it's important to know that. Although our lives may feel long at times, in a wider context they are just the blink of an eye, and it's imperative that we prioritize the right things while we can. I see too many people prioritizing financial status, job titles, salaries or how their CV looks over seeing the world, a well-deserved career break or even a sabbatical.

Nothing quite sums it up for me like this:

> 'So, of all your businesses, which did you like the most?'
>
> The answer took less than a second of thought. 'None of them.'
>
> He explained that he had spent more than 30 years with people he didn't like to buy things he didn't need. Life had become a succession of trophy wives – he was on lucky number three – expensive cars, and other empty bragging rights. Mark was one of the living dead.
>
> Timothy Ferriss, *The 4-Hour Work Week*

We must sit back and determine what we want from life. Do we actually want to be the CEO of a company, or just have the financial status to provide for a family and buy an overly pretentious SUV to drop the kids off at school in?

We must identify how these values may influence our state of mental health, too (which is always largely subjective). We have vegans on one side of the ongoing nutrition and wellness debate and carnivores on the other. But rarely do people ever sit back and think about the biological differences between one human and another. No one can truly be 'right' in a debate of this kind. Think about it this way: to one human a handful of peanuts is a snack, while to another it's a death sentence.

Starting a family or not is also a choice, although society and family pressure often push us in the direction of having children, and there is a sense of not having succeeded on some level if you don't toe the line (similar to the mortgage – see p. 153). It's like you failed the biological purpose of being a human if you decide not to have children, but this thinking overlooks one of the biggest given rights to humans: our prerogative. You can do as you like, based on your own values, not your parents' or anyone else's. How to decide? Well, go back to your values and correlate them with something important like state of mind: does having children benefit or negatively impact your values over time? What do you prioritize more in life?

Having children because you should is not the same as having children because you want to.

Working a job you dislike because you should is not the same as working a job because you want to.

There is no life you *should* or *have to* live, only the life you want to live – because, well, life is too short. Neil (deGrasse Tyson) has showed us that. If I remove societal pressures, my values involve being stress-free and in an environment that makes me happy. For that I must prioritize good weather, not doing things I don't like and eventually, one day, getting that dog. It just so happens I began writing this book very close to the beach and less than a thirty-minute drive to that steak restaurant I spoke about earlier.

The hard-to-swallow pill about your later life

Now, I'm going to ruffle your feathers with a point that you may not want to accept; you'll push back, and it's cool. I did, too, when I first thought about it. So, basically, when we look at our problems, we then use them as an excuse, a scapegoat for not doing what we want to in life. For instance, we see money as a problem: 'I'll do it when I have more money.' Or we talk about freedom or 'not having the time', almost as if in a few years' time there will be thirty hours in each day rather than twenty-four. Many of us are sitting waiting for the ideal life, right? That's what we're working towards each day. Let me guess: financial freedom, having the time to read each day, after meditating, that is, then we will travel, then we will have kids and then, and only then, we'll get a dog. We foresee a future that's easier than our present, and we do it naively and blindly, too. We assume there will be less stress, fewer responsibilities and we see the golden era of time to do things as being ahead of us, rather than with us right now.

More often than not, the reality is that we can do all of those things right now. We're just putting them off, waiting for a better time when we (falsely) think we won't have any problems in life. Merely a delay, merely excuse after excuse.

If you wait until you earn more money, you'll just stay in more expensive places when you travel.

If you wanted to read and meditate each day, you could, you'd just need to swap out a bit of your social-media time to do it.

If you really want a dog or to have kids, I'm sure if I put a gun to your head you'd make it work. You'd make it work great. So why should we need the gun?

Here's the big issue to me: the pressing elephant in the room.

Right now, we're all bang in the middle of the part of our lives we used to look forward to the most and all we're doing is putting things off, gambling in the hope for something better, and with no guarantee it's going to be that way. We put a pause on our aims, objectives, goals and dreams, waiting for the 'right time', when the stars will align. But the harsh reality is they probably won't and our situation will remain very much the same.

The answer here is realizing that you are in control and you are the one who must effect the changes that you want, which is pretty empowering.

> ### TASK
> The worst-case scenario isn't that bad. Play it out in your head. What's the silver lining that comes with it? Write it down, make it real. Make sure you put the worst-case scenario in lower case and the silver lining in capital letters. Look at your problems more as blessings: would you trade yours for anyone else's? I very much doubt it. Are you using your problems to hold yourself back from what you want to actually do in life? If you knew you'd go blind next year, what would you do tomorrow? If I put a gun to your head to do what you really wanted, would you do it? Ask yourself that every time you get excited about something in life. I do. I ask

myself all the time. We can accomplish what we want when we want. Waiting for the right time or the stars to align sounds like something the herd do – and we're not following them, are we?

If there is a feeling in your gut that you want to pursue a different career, then do it. Trust me on this, you'd much rather a life of tripping, failing and hustling within that thing you're passionate about than the constant feeling that you're not doing what you want to be doing, even if it feels like the easier option. This goes for leaving your partner too, I'm afraid, or starting the regime to finally get your shit together with training and nutrition. Unfortunately, when things are left unattended in life, they get worse, never better. When you sense toothache coming it's best to go see the dentist straight away. Be proactive whenever you feel the ache; it may not be pleasant, but if it's the right thing to do, then it must be done.

Future Anxiety

I once heard a definition of anxiety as 'worrying about things that may not even happen'. I find myself struggling with this most at airports before I travel. Perhaps slightly strangely, I see each day as being a bit like an experiment with many variables.* You will go through and compute very much the same experiences one day to the next, but you just may not know it yet. For instance, the café you go to: you know the quality of the coffee and the speed of the Wi-Fi, so when you decide to go back it's because the variables that suit your values are safe. To try a new coffee shop is to open up more variables; this could be beneficial, but could also come with risks.

I feel we human beings tend to like routine because it controls variables. When clients worried about weighing their food cooked vs raw, I'd tell that them as long as they did it the same each day it didn't matter, as the variables were kept the same. Whether they're correct or incorrect they're still consistent. When I travel, I experience anxiety I suppose because those variables are now taken out of my control: traffic on the way to the airport, a queue at security, my bag getting confiscated, mistaken identity or a cavity search. I am

* Every anxiety can be disabled or broken down into more digestible pieces. We just need to explore them a bit within each situation. It begins with why we feel that way and practising a bit of honesty with ourselves. These anxieties will often hold the weight we give them. It could be a date, a deadline or a financial problem. Either way, we need to simply weigh up the associated variables, the worst-case scenario and what the options are.

worrying about things that not only may not happen, they almost definitely won't.

We can't ignore 'future anxiety', though, and often if we try to, we can end up amplifying it further. So, what can we do? We can identify each anxiety factor and dissect it with pragmatic reasoning, giving it statistical weight. For instance, protecting ourselves from the uncontrollable traffic variable: we can check the travel times for that time of the day, leave early, creating a safe time buffer, choose a route or mode of transport we've used before. When looking at injured athletes returning to training, we look at risks vs rewards of returning a bit too early against a bit 'too late'. Implications of a bit too early – injury again; 'too late' actually means even more chance for a full or even fuller recovery, saving time in the long run.

I was an army cadet when I was younger, and I'll never forget the saying: 'If you can't be on time, be early'. Being early can help reduce anxiety, but what else? Well, personally, I make a mental or written list of exactly what is making me anxious. If it's about what's in my backpack, I'll do a search to check what could be in there that's not allowed, and I'll do my due diligence. These things can strategically reduce 'future anxiety'.

Again, I am not telling you how to make future anxiety go away, but instead how to manage it, how to reduce its impact on your mind. It's not about ignoring or suppressing emotions; it's about recognizing them, giving them weight or even making them real on a bit of paper.

TASK

Is there any action you can take to reduce the weight of that anxiety on your mind? What would that action be? Write it down. How would that action reduce the anxiety? Maybe keep a notes section in your phone for things such as 'Airport travel', 'First date', 'Presentation', 'Asking for a promotion'. Identify the key factors that are making you anxious – spelling mistakes, areas you may struggle to explain or even appearance. Something as simple as double-checking your spelling or ensuring that your flies aren't undone can eradicate that anxiety and increase confidence.

Before moving on, I want to be honest with you: I don't deal with my anxiety alone. I have a very good friend named Lucy who has single-handedly armed me with the tools I need to manage it. I asked her, 'If you had a thousand words, what would you share?' And here it is:

Mark Twain once famously said, 'I've had a lot of worries in my life, most of which never happened'; much like sitting in a rocking chair, anxiety gives us something to do, but doesn't actually get us anywhere. For some people, it's fleeting and for others (myself included) anxiety can sometimes feel like an Internet browser with twenty-three tabs open, two frozen and no idea where the music is coming from. A constant hum of impending doom, anxiety can negatively affect everything from your sleep, productivity and eating habits to relationships and general ability to find joy and ease in day-to-day life. Coupled with nausea and a racing heartbeat that feels like your brain is swelling and sounds like somebody is using your eardrums as a giant gong, being caught up in the anxiety cycle is not a very pleasant place to be. The good news is, it isn't something that you have to just 'learn to live with'.

Anxiety is a normal, healthy and expected emotion experienced by everyone in some form; first-date butterflies, waiting for doctor's results, me after three consecutive coffees. Managing 'future anxiety' by controlling the variables that we have power over – making an effort to arrive early, practising activities that promote a calmer headspace, me *not* having three consecutive coffees – can certainly make a big difference, though there are two practices in particular that I have found to have a profound effect on the disordered and constant sense that something bad is going to happen.

The stoic exercise *'premeditatio malorum'* (premeditation of evils) is one in which you actively think about things that could go wrong or be taken away from you, and plan what you would do in those cases. Why the fuck would you do that, I hear you ask? Because it stares anxiety straight in the face. Rather than running from it or hiding behind the distractions so readily available in the modern world, we metaphorically pull up a chair and invite the anxiety to take a seat. Like an investigator, we become curious about it. What does it feel like? Where do you feel it? What are you afraid of? Failure, feeling inadequate, making a fool of yourself, other people's opinions, losing something or someone? What is the worst thing that could happen – no, really: *the worst thing*? Should that happen (and it's probably useful to point out at this stage that 95 per cent of the time, it doesn't happen at all, or only to a much lesser extent) what would you do?

In *The 4-Hour Work Week*, author Timothy Ferris credits his similarly stoic-inspired exercise of 'fear setting' with being the most valuable one he does. Sir Richard Branson, the self-made billionaire, entrepreneur and founder of the Virgin Group, writes in his book *Losing*

My Virginity about the importance of 'protecting the downside'. Once Branson had negotiated the price for his first second-hand 747 from Boeing, he made a plan that if Virgin Atlantic wasn't successful, he'd be able to hand the plane back after the first year. Protecting the downside is looking at any situation and determining all options before making a decision, so that we can identify the worst-case scenario and work backwards from there to find the optimal route forwards. What I have found with this exercise is that regardless of the fear or root cause of my anxiety – a potentially career-ruining decision, a financial investment which puts everything at risk, looking bad in front of my peers, letting someone (or myself) down – the worst-case scenario usually involves at least one of the following: pain, disappointment, financial loss, discomfort, heartbreak and a giant bruise to the ego. But that's about it. Hindsight would even lead me to believe that when things do go wrong (which they do) this can, in fact, be a recipe for building resilience: a chance to give it another go, start from scratch or move in another direction, with more experience, humility and patience – and a lot less ego.

By planning for the absolute worst and considering your options should that scenario ever come to pass, you've got no more to worry about.

> *We are more often frightened than hurt; and we suffer more*
> *from imagination than from reality.*
>
> Seneca

Of course, failure is not only inevitable, it is essential. It's our actions after the event of failing that matter the most. Learning how to 'fail forward' could be the most powerful yet underused practice we have at our disposal.

The second exercise is to reframe the anxiety with an opposing question. 'What if it all goes wrong?' Well, what if it all goes right? 'What if I lose money?' becomes 'What if I make money?' 'What if they don't like me?' 'What if they do?' It's funny that when our anxious minds grab on to something negative, we can create endless warped stories of all the bad things that might happen, but when we flip it round with a positive, it doesn't work the same way. Instead, we are left with a blank space, a brief (but blissful) feeling of relief and, for me, the image of a monkey scratching its head. Psychologists refer to this as a negativity bias, and it is our brain's natural tendency to ruminate on negative possibilities rather than positive ones. By recognizing the anxiety and reframing it – 'What happens if it all works out?' – we start to loosen the shackles on our minds. We interrupt the vicious washing-machine-on-full-spin anxiety cycle and, when practised over time, much like hypertrophy in a muscle, our ability to more positively question our anxiety becomes stronger. This is known as brain neuroplasticity: the brain's ability to adapt to change with repetition of a thought or emotion when we reinforce neural pathways, a technique often used in cognitive behavioural therapy. When we change the way we think, we change the way we feel.

Anxiety, at best, can be a normal, intermittent and expected human experience. At worst, chronic, irrational and persistent anxiety can trap us in fear and hold us back from ever realizing our true potential. By recognizing and becoming curious about our anxiety, we can disarm it and start to dissolve its destructive power.

Lucy Lord, @lordlucy

Dating

You may not be interested in dating. You may have found the one – or *wahid* (meaning one in Arabic). I joke with friends, saying we're searching for the 'wahid'. In fact, one of my favourite things in recent years has been discovering the countries where Arabic is spoken – up to twenty-five, I believe. The majority of English people have this thing where we expect everyone else to speak English, but through having friends from all kinds of multicultural backgrounds, I've made a conscious effort to learn some of their languages. Whether I'm at dinner with someone from Egypt or ordering something from a Moroccan restaurant, sometimes saying '*mashallah*' as a way of showing appreciation can really surprise people and bring a smile to their faces. Even if you get it completely wrong and say it in the wrong context, you'll probably still make people smile.

But back to dating. I don't mean to bring a negative into the situation, but I want to mention that everyone who gets married thinks it's because they've found the person they'll spend a lifetime with. Yet 42 per cent of marriages in the UK end in divorce, so it's my inner pragmatist and not the pessimist bringing you this section. People will date, even people who are married now can still potentially have dates in the future, that's my point. If your marriage is one of the successful ones, then maybe give this advice to someone who may need it.

There are a lot of things that I think are wrong in the world and one of them is dating and how most people go about it. In essence, we're just much more organized and tame versions of dogs sniffing bums as we go past someone that we find interesting or attractive. Dating, going for a drink or even a meal is the ultimate bum sniff. The majority of grafting is often done in the build-up on social-media dating apps to ensure we're not walking into a metaphorical ambush. But what are most people striving for, ultimately? I'd say compatibility.

One of the best changes I made to my life in the last couple of years was to no longer go on 'first dates' as they're known traditionally.

> *A person's success in life can usually be measured*
> *by the number of uncomfortable conversations*
> *he or she is willing to have.*
>
> Timothy Ferriss, *The 4-Hour Work Week*

Dates often make people very anxious, and the drop-out rate can be very high, where people cancel last minute, mostly through fear, using an excuse such as 'something has come up'. Some people take it to heart, but maybe the other person was just a bit scared and that is normal. Being 'stood up' is a well-known thing and I think anxiety more than anything is the culprit.

I've often got caught up in my emotions and 'worst-case scenarios' when it comes to dating: 'What if we have nothing to talk about and sit in silence waiting for food?' 'What if they don't look anything like their app pictures?'

I'd say from personal experience that if a date is called off, it's at the last minute, when someone takes their friend's unsolicited advice to heart or they feel too anxious about the outcome and many other factors. This is where my tactic comes in: the fifteen-minute date.

Fifteen minutes is more than long enough for both parties to have an adequate bum sniff (pardon my crass nature). There are many variations to this dating process. You can include a dog or a planned after-work walk. I will often ask someone if they want to have a dip in the sea or grab an ice cream. Even sharing a walk to a Tube station or through a park of choice. Who doesn't have fifteen minutes? Who doesn't like ice cream? (If they don't like ice cream, that's a certain red flag in my eyes; if they do like ice cream, but opt for a cup over a cone, that's also risky territory.) And who doesn't want to meet a dog for a short walk? There's no pressure, no dress code, you can forget your perfume or aftershave. You might think I sound like a fucking robot, but sometimes removing something from context and calling it what it is can help the situation.

And I find the best part is this: if you're not interested and you don't talk much after, it's very hard to be considered a dickhead who never texted after a first date. Instead, you're just the person they shared a dip in the sea or a walk around the park with. Time is often wasted on first dates, money, too, and if they go badly, they increase anxiety around the next time. This can mean that someone's dating 'pipeline' (if you were to think of it as being a bit like sales) would remain barren and empty, increasing their chances of getting back with an ex and never finding the 'wahid'.

> *They're your ex for a reason.*
>
> James Smith

Also, if you go on five dates a week, you're not going to have much time to see your friends, have much-needed alone time or masturbate near enough to your requirements. However, fifteen-minute dates? Easy. I once needed to get a T-shirt for a night out, so I invited a girl I'd never met to come give me a hand. She thought I was peculiar; I told her the deal. I bought her a coffee and we had a right laugh as I picked the T-shirt. Instead of sitting in an interview-style dating scenario obvious from the outside to others,* we were mooching around shops and having a laugh. I said I'd take her for a proper dinner at the end of the date, and I opted to wear the T-shirt we'd chosen together.

Realistically, if you had three fifteen-minute meets per week as opposed to one date night, you'd save money and time, you'd reduce your anxiety and you'd increase the likelihood of finding someone who is compatible. I have yet to find a downside to the fifteen-minute date, and paired with the sleep you save from not getting drunk in order to endure the bland nature of a bad date you are really on to a winner. It may not be for everyone, but it's certainly worth trying out.

On the flipside, it's worth noting that it's important to have time alone, too. That's general advice for those who are looking for a partner. I love reminding people of this:

A crowded world thinks that aloneness is always loneliness and that to seek it is perversion.

John Graves

---

* When dating after the initial fifteen-minute meet and you lock in the dinner or drinks, don't sit opposite the person if you have the option. Sitting beside someone has a better feel, so opt for booths or even a communal table to remove the interview-esque feel. Also, doing things that you would do with a partner is a great date idea. You get to try before you buy what it'd be like to date them, which is very fitting in itself. When personal training I had a few tricks up my sleeve to make the client comfortable in our first sessions. I'd ask them, 'What coffee do you want?' rather than asking if they wanted one and I'd often get them to carry my water bottle around the gym for me, so it felt like we'd been training together a lot longer. Use this on dates. Be creative and don't follow the herd's idea of a date. Keep in mind, if you matched this person on a dating app, they're no doubt talking to other people, so appear unique and pick something rogue now and then. When everyone else is asking for 'a drink' you could invite them rock climbing instead. Punchy, yet effective.

Let's not mistake the two. It's important to have time to yourself to reflect, empty the mind and to just enjoy your own company. A good book and some time alone can be a powerful contributor to having a clear mind and the mental-health benefits that come with it.

To conclude: don't overcommit to dating, and make it work for both parties. Being in a relationship versus being single is a two-sided coin. There will be times in either scenario when you wish for the other, so whatever situation you're in, enjoy it.

Regression to the Mean

What if I told you that I thought the majority of performance-related feedback was more often than not absolutely fucking useless?

Let's imagine I take you to play bowls on a sunny day in Sydney. You have no previous bowling experience. You throw down a white ball to begin – this is called a 'jack', from the Latin word *jactus*, meaning a cast or a throw (sorry, I can't help it – I'm on my own journey of discovery writing this book, so it's only fair you join me). How will your first bowl go? No one knows, but let me tell you this:

- ► If you do very well the first bowl, your next will do worse.
- ► If you do very poorly the first bowl, your next will do better.
- ► However, your skill set at the given task will remain very much the same.

This is regression to the mean (the mean being a calculated 'central' value of a set of numbers), which we touched on earlier. Now, when you do poorly first time around, I could give you an arbitrary piece of advice for you to improve (and I'd get gratification for my incredible skills). If it's the other way around, I'd probably say you got a bit too cocky with your second one and needed to do what you did the first time around. You'd need to bowl hundreds of times to determine an accurate 'mean' positioning. When we look at 10,000 hours of mastery I very much doubt someone's performance is really influenced by a single bowl.

Should I have a poor performance training in Brazilian jiu jitsu, statistically speaking I'll probably do better in my next session. Should I dominate above normal, chances are it will return back to the mean. Of course it will; that's life. That's also maths. I like to think the same about most high days and low days: on a low day, I can sit and think that it will at some point regress to the mean. On high days, the same – I know it's short lived. We experience this with trauma and huge successes in life, too: cloud nine won't last for ever; our minds will not permit it. So, if I come to your house with your dream car, I can guarantee that within three months you will be bored of it. Conversely, if someone close to you dies – I don't wish it, of course, but in three months you'll be on your way back to the mean.

Depression is when that mean is a lot lower than it should be. This can be, as mentioned earlier, due to a genetic predisposition, but it can also be from environment, stress, toxic relationships, etc.

It's like I said earlier on in the book about those world-class models – how someone somewhere is already bored of sleeping with them. Again, it's regression to the mean, returning to the norm. With any change above or below performance, mood or emotions there will be a return to normal (see References, p. 256):

Regression toward (or to) the mean is the phenomenon that arises if a random variable is extreme on its first measurement but closer to the mean or average on its second measurement and if it is extreme on its second measurement but closer to the average on its first.

To avoid making incorrect inferences, regression toward the mean must be considered when designing scientific experiments and interpreting data.

I think it's important to remember that when we're low we will come back; when we're great, vice versa. The mean, over time, is governed by us, our environment and who we surround ourselves with, and rather than looking for instances of extreme happiness, we should instead look for lifestyle changes that will shift the mean to a better position. Being consistent with training would increase your mean performance; consistency with diet and lifestyle would benefit your mean health; and ensuring management of stress, sunlight and relationships would hugely benefit the mean positioning of your mental health.

Why is it that people believe in luck? The lottery, for example, one in millions and they actually believe there's a chance they can win. Yet with maths it's overlooked. If you kicked a football at a goal there is a statistical number of times it will go in per person – that's a fact, not a belief. Now, to improve that number requires training. Over time, some will miss and some will go in; only repeating the process will benefit your 'mean' score over time. I want you to think the same about job interviews and the same about asking someone out. You have a 'mean' score already and when things don't work out that's part of the maths, it's part of life.

When throwing darts at a dart board, one may miss the target alto-gether and get stuck in the wall, but you don't give up and never play with your friends again. So, I need you to appreciate that occasionally things will go wrong – the interview will end terribly, the person whose number you ask for won't speak English – but you have to brush it off and continue because it's just an anomaly around the mean. It takes hundreds of repetitions to figure out where you sit, how your accuracy is, but the good isn't the good without the bad – and without both we can't have this average.

It can seem daunting at first, but trust me on this: when we repeat-edly do something, it's not to hit the bullseye every time. Quite the opposite. It's to repeat and repeat to improve the overall average, to shift the mean to an improved position. If you start asking people out, your mean may only be that one in five says yes. Over time, through asking, that number will improve. And before you know it, your mean will be two in five.

No one is better than you. They just may have a better 'mean' score, because they're probably further down the line of practising, and that's fine. We don't need to have the best score, just the desired outcome from whatever it is that we do. We must anticipate missing and anticipate doing better than expected. Some days will go much better, while others will no doubt go a lot worse, but things will always make their way back to the average.

Trust in your own abilities not only to succeed, but to fail, too. See failure as a stepping stone to improving your overall score over time, not looking for singular wins but instead a spread of more accurate shots in life. Do not put your blind faith in luck – put it in yourself and the belief that you have the tools you need to quit the job you hate and pursue whatever it is you want to do. If the dart misses the target, don't feel bad about it. Why would you? Think about it this way: if you throw a really bad shot, statistically speaking the next one is going to be better, much better – that's not a pep talk, that's maths. So, smile, appreciate that you missed and be confident the next one will be better. Chances are that it will be.

Real-Life Learning

I spoke briefly about Brazilian jiu jitsu in my first book, but it is now such a big part of my life that I think the sport needs a bit more of the limelight. There are so many lessons to learn from it – all the way from humility to respect and discipline. You may or may not be in a position to take it up, but if it was up to me, I'd make it compulsory in schools. The respect element is very similar to rugby – it's very physical, but everyone has the utmost respect for their opponents, and although people can get hurt, it's not the objective.

Lessons to learn from jiu jitsu

If you ever got into a fight with a boxer, you would walk away in pretty bad shape. If you got into a fight with a jiu-jitsu practitioner, chances are you'd leave without a mark or wound on your body. The sport is about controlling and rendering your opponent useless without hurting them. It's a big part of mixed martial arts and known as the 'ground component' of combative fighting. The sport is growing and being used by everyone from bouncers to the police to restrain people while keeping both parties safe. A black belt is the highest grade, and you're easily looking at a decade of full-time commitment for that. I've seen some of the toughest men in the world break down and cry when they receive their black belt, and it's something I very much hope to achieve one day.

Your first day in the gym you're given your white belt, and there are no stripes on it. Each time you 'grade', you're given a stripe to signify your progression. There are four stripes allocated before the next promotion. From your white belt you progress to blue, then purple, then brown, then black. They say it's about two years of hard work for each belt; if you're a bit half-arsed, it could take you easily four to six years per belt. I love the idea of 'always being a white belt' – meaning that no matter where you are in life, you're a student of something. I had 100,000 followers but no stripe on my white belt. No financial standing or follower status can help you when the four lowest-grade students get the buckets out and wipe the mats. I remember the first time I had to wipe down the sweat on the mats, thinking that this was an environment I could learn a lot from – not just the combative nature of the sport, but the knowledge that you can always learn from others. You may think you're at the top, but all it takes is to walk into another gym and someone else will be better, will have trained harder and be more ready than you are for the 'roll', as it's called. You could be a janitor or a CEO in your white belt, but no matter what, you keep your feet clean, shoes off the mat and at the end, you tie your belt, bow to each training companion and shake hands with everyone who just tried to kill you.

The rules are complex yet simple. You begin standing. The idea is to get your opponent on the floor where they are a lot less of a threat to you. Even the likes of Mike Tyson are less threatening on the floor. (In jiu jitsu, they say the floor is the water in which many cannot swim, and the experts are the sharks that prey in it.) Takedowns to the floor will secure you two points, so if nothing else happens in the match, you'll win from those two points alone. Once your opponent is on the floor, there's every chance they'll use their legs to defend themselves. This is what occurs in most street fights, so it's important to make sure the legs don't cause you any issues. In jiu jitsu, when your opponent is on the floor and their legs are in between you and them, it's known as their 'guard'. You are permitted to pass it however you like without striking your opponent, as there is no striking in jiu jitsu. If you manage to 'pass the guard' of your opponent, you are granted another three points. (I know all this can sound complex, but understanding it could be the difference between you trying and not trying jiu jitsu, and as it's one of the best decisions I have ever made in my life, I think it's still worthy of a detailed explanation.)

Once you have passed the guard of your opponent through blunt force, sly tactics, misdirection or being cunning, you'll end up in some form of 'pin'. In wrestling, the idea is to pin the opponent on their back and the entire sport revolves around that one pin, but in jiu jitsu we have several. You may secure a mounted position (four points), you may get into 'side control' or even 'knee on belly' (two points) – each position can get you access to the next, all depending on your own game plan. You're allocated points for the most offensive; taking your opponent's back is the most sought-after position, scoring the same as the mount (four points). At any point from the first second to the last you can attempt a submission – this is to make your opponent submit, by saying the word 'tap' loudly. This is especially handy when your hands are unable to tap physically – any yell of any kind will count as a submission. The idea is not to hurt your opponent, but to put pressure on a joint or choke to get your win. If there are no submissions, the person who was dominant through point accumulation wins.

Training in jiu jitsu is unique. In rugby or boxing, training is only an exercise in honing your skills – as a boxer you spend most of your time against pads, a mirror and punch bags, not an actual opponent. In football and even rugby, it's usually a case of drills and fitness with a mix of game plays, and 'live' training is limited. In jiu jitsu, in most classes there is sparring or 'rolling', where you're permitted to go as hard as you like (I mentioned *porrada* in *Not a Diet Book*, whereby you respect your opponent at all times, but you never give them an easy ride); you can't be letting them think life is easy when they leave the gym.

You trim your nails, observe good hygiene, wait for permission to stand on the mat; you shake everyone's hand, you bow before you roll and there is a hierarchy of respect.

We stand in order of belts to begin and end each session. It doesn't matter who you are, if a billionaire starts jiu jitsu he will wipe the mats with the other white belts, he will stand in line at the bottom of the food chain and we'll probably share a laugh as I help him remember how to tie his belt properly.

Your first six months resemble drowning: you know what is happening, but there is not much you can do about it. You just have to keep turning up, keep giving it everything and keep losing. In your spare time, you become a student – hungry to learn what happened to you in your last roll, what you can do to escape that position in future – and you just hope that the next time your training partner decides to fold your clothes you're not still wearing them. You train in two sets of clothing, 'Gi' and 'No Gi', and compete in either one or the other. Your Gi is your kimono, which resembles your mum's dressing gown, and I suppose it's to mimic what happens in self-defence when people grab your clothes. Having grips on your opponent means you can not only control distance, but your opponent, and they can do the same back to you. Your collar can be used to choke you and even your lapel in the wrong hands can cause all kinds of trouble. No Gi is usually in shorts and a rash guard; no grabbing of clothes is permitted. If you've ever trained judo, where your objective is to get your opponent on the floor for an ippon,* you'll prefer Gi to begin with.

If you did wrestling at high school, you'll prefer No Gi to begin with, I am sure. It's about changes in height levels and aggressive shooting towards the legs for takedowns where you can attempt to score with a pin.

Should I have children, I couldn't imagine a better sport for them to learn to defend themselves. Not only would they pick up some good techniques for cleaning the floor thoroughly, most importantly they would learn respect for a hierarchy not defined by money, fame or status but instead by hard work and consistency.

TASK

Google your closest jiu-jitsu gym and consider getting your white belt. There is no age or size limit or any other barrier. Jean Jacques Machado, for example, is one of the most highly regarded black belts in the world. So much so that he is one of the few people on Earth to wear a coral belt, which is black and red. He was born with a birth defect known as amniotic band syndrome (meaning one of his hands was deformed, leaving him with just a thumb and little finger on one hand).

There are some days when I find it tough, and I'm tired, deflated and struggling, but I just think about that person out there who has it harder than me who isn't complaining about it. The toughest thing of all is to just turn up. I never leave a session wishing I hadn't been.

---

* Ippon is the highest score in judo, awarded for a throw that places the opponent on their back with impetus or for holding the opponent on their back for a number of seconds.

> You may love the sport, or you may want to do Muay Thai or boxing instead, but just begin something – begin the journey of 'always being a white belt'. Remember Carol Dweck's words quoted earlier: 'becoming is better than being'.

New skills and training anxiety

I bet as soon as you consider the idea of starting a new sport you're hit with training anxiety. And guess what? It's normal. I'm a very experienced personal trainer, but when I use a gym for the first time, I'm anxious – even more so than the average person sometimes. I walk over to a complex-looking leg press and I think: James, you've been training people for nearly a decade – you should know how this leg press works. I jump on like Sherlock Holmes and try to figure it out; not that long ago I got on a leg extension at my local gym only to realize shortly afterwards it was a hamstring curl. No one was looking, though, and I got away without the embarrassment! But the point I want to make clear here is how normal this is. We all feel this way. We all feel like the entire world is watching when we exercise and when we train. I remember an experiment where students walked into classes late and were asked to guess how many people noticed their tardiness.* It turned out that they hugely overestimated the number who noticed them. And we do this everywhere in life: when we trip up in public, knock a drink over or turn up anywhere late – we feel all eyes are on us,

* Tardiness: the quality or fact of being late; lateness. And I've included this footnote because I only learned this word when writing this book.

but often it's just human nature and no one really cares, as they're too caught up in how late they are or spilling their own drink.

I don't think there is really any way to avoid the anxiety we face when training in a new or even a known environment. Instead, we must just deal with it, but also appreciate it. And the reason I say that is because we all require some degree of anxiety to perform well. (See References, p. 256.)

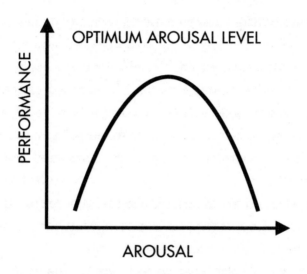

This is known as the inverted U hypothesis and is one of the most interesting things I remember learning in college. I will be the first to put my hand up and say that there is a mixed bag of studies surrounding this, so let's stick with identifying it as a hypothesis. However, from a personal, anecdotal standpoint, I am very grateful for a lot of the anxiety I feel in situations because of this hypothesis. This upside down 'U' is different for everyone, but I think it certainly exists. Let me give you some examples.

I'm playing rugby and my dream has finally come true – my coach has said, 'Smithy, you're kicking for goal.' If this was at Twickenham stadium, in front of a packed crowd of 80,000, nerves, tremors and doubt would sweep my mind and I'd be much more concerned about the thousands of onlookers than the kick for goal. On the other hand, if I was at Maheno RFC in North Otago, New Zealand, where I played in 2012, it would be another story. I spent a season playing rugby in the South Island of New Zealand and I was positioned in Maheno, where the population of the town was seventy-five people. In the wider district there were six rugby teams among 10,000 people, the clubs of three of which shared the same car park. On a good day, the neighbouring sheep outnumbered the onlookers three to one, and there would be a substantial reduction in anxiety brought on by onlookers. Under the gaze of the sheep, I may have been on the other end of the spectrum, namely underaroused (not like that) – I could be almost blasé, as the kick wouldn't matter quite so much. So, I would need the perfect level of anxiety to match my personality for optimal performance.

I've experienced this at golf, too. On the range we're hitting them like Tiger Woods, but as soon as we get to the first hole we bend it like Beckham and beg our friends to let us go again.

A more likely situation may be seen with a marathon runner: too many onlookers and they may be out the gates too fast and experience fatigue too early, burning out before the halfway mark. On the flip side, they may perform a trial run with no onlookers and go too slow because of the lack of pressure, crossing the line with fuel in the tank and without the result they expected.

This theory was proposed by psychologists Yerkes and Dodson in 1908, so it's been around for a pretty long time. Then in 1943, the 'Drive Reduction Theory' was developed – a linear model of the inverted U going from bottom left to top right in a straight line. This supported the idea that the more aroused the athlete is, the better their performance, but I don't agree with that. I've seen basketball players go to shit aiming for buzzer shots as the game time runs out. And we regularly see big mistakes made in soccer penalty shootouts, so I can't get behind that hypothesis, nor any, in fact, that stipulates 'more is better'.

When any research is conducted on negative emotions it is no surprise that there is a lot of focus on anxiety. This is largely to do with the fact that anxiety negatively impacts mental health for a lot of people around the world each day. It's probably a key reason why there is so much focus on its impact on sports performance.

Based on meta analysis (the examination) of multiple studies, there is typically a negative relationship between anxiety and sporting performances. (See References, p. 256.) Although, as of more recently, it is understood that having little to no anxiety leading up to and during a competition can also be detrimental to an athlete's performance. (See References, p. 256.) **Therefore, it's all about the sweet spot.**

If we can get into the mindset that some anxiety is welcome in certain training environments, I think it makes the entire management aspect of it so much easier to come to terms with. Going to a new gym, for example, and therefore leaving your comfort zone is good. If you were to feel no anxiety, it could be to your detriment. Game day. Feeling the nerves? Good, you need them. Feeling nothing would be the flip side and no one wants that.

To conclude, try to embrace that feeling and know that other people feel it, too. The only way you're going to get comfortable with whatever is in front of you – whether it's a confusing leg press or a new martial-arts gym – is to remember: no harm in giving it a go, and I'm sure someone will always be willing to help.

Always a white belt

Everyone on this planet learns from experience – that's a no brainer. Whether it's touching something hot when you're younger and always being cautious afterwards, eating ice cream too fast or running on a slippery surface, it's fair to say that human beings learn from their own experiences. **But not everyone can learn from other people's experiences.** When you learn from other people's experiences you can accomplish so much more in much less time. I'll never forget a few years back, I was doing a live video on Facebook in which I told everyone about my business idea: the James Smith Academy. About an hour later, I got an email from a complete stranger and all it said was, 'Before you start your business idea, read this book.' It was called *Zero to One* by Peter Thiel (the co-founder of PayPal).

> *All failed companies are the same:*
> *they failed to escape competition.*
>
> Peter Thiel, *Zero to One: Notes on Startups,*
> *or How to Build the Future*

I came to realize one thing: that I actually did not want to compete with anyone. I decided to learn from failed businesses, to use their bad experience to ensure I didn't take the same steps. This was my first business, and I decided to boldly move down a path to compete with absolutely no one. Of course, this seems mad and I have been asked hundreds of times: 'How do you train people online?' Well, you provide the same solutions to the same problems through technology instead of face to face. I think our egos can often want us to start up shop to just 'do better' than other people. That finite mindset again. We'd rather beat them than be truly innovative in a new space where we compete with … well, no one.

Books can be a tool to learn from other people's experiences, their ups and their downs. Their mistakes and their successes, their good ideas and their bad ones. To proactively learn from other people's mistakes is what can make the difference between being good and being great. Michael Jordan would notoriously study the players he came up against in the NBA. Whether your passion is running a basket-weaving business or selling services, someone somewhere can teach you lessons about their own mistakes. It takes a huge amount of humility to realize that you're a student and that you can learn from every encounter. Every person you meet can teach you something valuable and every culture can, too. Whoever can tie their imaginary white belt the most in situations will take away the most from the encounter.

Let's take being a student in martial arts, for instance. When a boxer tells you to keep your gloves up when you throw a punch it's proba-bly because they've made that mistake too many times and taken a few blows to the chin because of it. One thing I find is that highly experienced coaches don't just say stuff for the sake of it; they say it because they're passionate about what they're doing and it's impera-tive you listen. I'll never forget in my office days one of the owners of the business who, if I had to describe him in one word, I'd say he was 'wise'. He would lean back in his chair and talk to prospects incredibly slowly, leaving long pauses to let the other person speak. And he'd always say to me, 'James, you have two ears and only one mouth for a reason.' This is about listening more than you speak, which for me is a hard thing, as I do love the sound of my own voice here and there! But I do listen, too. When a black belt in jiu jitsu tells you not to put your hand somewhere, it's not for the sake of hearing their own voice but usually from the experience of having done it themselves. If you can listen and if you can learn, you can skip the mistake they made at one time in their past.

There are so many days when I wake up and I don't want to go to training. I may feel sore, tired or just deflated from getting my arse handed to me the night before, but I think to myself: what one thing could I learn today? And I am not just saying this for the sake of this book; I have often dragged myself to training to end up learning something very simple, which has come along to save me when competing in front of dozens of people. And this is not limited to just sport – it applies to every avenue of life. Listen, learn, then try it out. What do you have to lose from someone else's experience?

People always want a mentor, someone to guide them, a life coach or a business coach, but I find that it's not so much a sensei we actually need, but the feeling of being a student and the humility that comes with knowing you don't know that much at all. I don't have a business coach, but going to training and occasionally being physically shown how low I am in the food chain has tremendously positive effects on my business, my relationships and how I approach life. And this doesn't have to be within a contact sport; it could be a language, a hobby, it could even be spending your spare time learning how to basket weave for all I care – but be a student. This is the direction to go in, rather than seeking a life coach who is probably only going to recycle mantras they've heard from someone else.

If I wasn't a student in some form, I think I'd feel a lot more lost in life, to be honest. For years, before jiu jitsu, I was learning about anatomy and mechanics, and every day I'd be challenged by a client I saw on the gym floor in some way. There weren't many days when I didn't learn, and I kept a notes page open on my phone at all times whenever I was challenged on something I didn't know. (Every martial artist reading this will be nodding their head in agreement now.) So, I want you too to become a student in the coming weeks in whatever you decide.

Have you ever realized that the majority of people who participate in contact sports aren't violent, they aren't thugs? They are, in fact, humble students who enjoy the process more than the outcome. They may not even know it, but they enjoy becoming more than being. A growth mindset without even realizing it.

Just because you're a good student with two ears doesn't mean you're a know it all, though. Being able to say you don't know something is also hugely important. What do you think sounds better: bullshitting your way in a subject you're not well informed on or saying, 'Look, I'm not actually sure of that answer; I'm going to make a note of it on my phone and next time I see you we can discuss it.' I spent lunch breaks and even the time driving to and from work listening to podcasts on the subjects in that notes field. One day, I was asked about how the menstrual cycle influenced performance and fat loss, and I had no idea, so I said, 'I honestly don't know.' But then I went away and read, looked at studies, listened to podcasts and discovered all I could on the subject. Before you knew it, I had a viral video on Facebook getting millions of views on a subject I'd known nothing about only a few weeks before. Just saying you don't know triggers your inner student to become inquisitive.

I personally don't consider myself to be very smart or intelligent, but I do see myself as being very **open to learning**, and that's what being a student is about.

Another area I really think is important to learn from is culture. I was hugely ignorant about culture for so long, thinking that being different was some kind of barrier between people. In the last few years, I have become friends with a Turkish Kurd and a Muslim, but I had no idea about what either of those things meant until I asked them to teach me about it.

To support my friend in Ramadan, I fasted with him so that we could enjoy our first meal together. What a learning experience it was! A younger, more ignorant version of myself would have considered the entire thing 'daft' and I'd have said something like. 'What's the point?' But although I only joined him for a fortnight, I completely understood the appreciation that comes with giving something up, how it brought us both closer together at the evening feeding window. I got a new and completely different perspective on it.

With Diren, I try to learn Turkish words to use with his parents, I try to understand their politics and I have so much respect for how close the family are and how there are so many similarities in our values, although our cultures are so different. I came to realize that if we all just took a closer look, we could be less ignorant than we are.

I don't come armed with a solution to racism or discrimination between cultures, but I do see a lot of ignorance, especially from white British people (like myself). Ignorance doesn't make you a bad person; it's just one of those things we must acknowledge. I always say that there are two types of people in the world: those who love cricket and those who don't understand it yet. I'm not comparing racism to cricket, but I feel that if we all understood each other's cultures a bit better there would be fewer divisions between us. Whether the Qur'an or the Bible or no religion at all, we all want the same things in life: to be treated well, spend time in families we love and to enjoy life. We share more than we think. After all, as I said earlier, birds flying in formation reduce drag – and that's irrespective of their breed or colour. Get my drift?

I admire cultures in Europe where people are a lot more honest and blunt, such as in the Netherlands and Germany. Having been shown to our room in a hotel in Berlin, I asked the hotel worker if the restaurant over the road was a good place to grab a bite to eat. He looked at me, smiled, then said, 'No.' Why use thirty words when one will do? We British are very guilty of doing the opposite: 'Well, I've only been there a few times and the food is nice, but I could think of some better places if you're looking for somewhere to go for dinner this evening.' I like directness and I think that if you were to spend enough time in Germany or Amsterdam you could become a lot better at saying no and declining things you don't want to do. British culture to me is about agreeing to meet up with someone you can't be arsed to catch up with because you're more worried about hurting their feelings than you are about your day, or being too polite to complain when a restaurant gets your order wrong, as you 'don't want to make a scene'. We can learn so much from other people. It seems such a big shame to only learn from our own experiences.

If you can read, you have the opportunity to excel beyond most by learning from the mistakes of people you may never meet. To neglect this opportunity to me is to limit your learning, which puts nothing between you and someone who *can't* read. Food for thought.

Reversing Emotions and Bias

There are many spectrums of light the human eye cannot see, but it doesn't mean they're not there – it merely requires a certain lens. For instance, you may be insecure about how many previous partners your lover has had, and that's an insecurity that plays on your mind all the time. You're afraid to ask, afraid to hear the answer. But it can be flipped: instead of fearing that 'a tiger never changes its stripes', you could think that someone who got busy early on in life could actually have it 'out of their system'. This is something to put your mind at ease – but only if you choose to put it at ease. Ultimately, you can't control or influence how many partners your lover has had, but you can control how you feel about it. There are other cases of turning one emotion into another. For instance, insecurities can be turned into gratitude when viewed through the right mental lens.

We are all more biased than we like to believe. I expect we're even biased about our own levels of bias. (That feels like something out of the film *Inception*.) Just as a reminder, our confirmation bias derives from our nature to 'search for, interpret, favour and recall information that confirms or supports one's prior personal beliefs or values'. Now, something I feel we don't like to acknowledge is that our prior experiences also govern our current bias. For instance, if you have had a partner in the past who cheated on you, when your current partner doesn't text back for a while you could think they're up to no good. That's an insecurity based solely on your own bias of previous experiences. Although it could be true, it's best that you reverse the bias by simply recognizing how the thought or notion has come to exist. Everyone has a bias and it's why jurors exist within the legal system: to bring a fresh set of eyes into the fray with no prior experience of (therefore no bias towards) the defendant. Whenever we get to a conclusion it's good to spend a fraction of a second determining how we got there and also whether we are letting a bias from a previous experience interfere with pragmatic thinking.

The attractiveness bias

What if I told you that if you're really good looking you'll spend less time in jail? Crazy to believe, and I'll explain more in a second, but before you get worried, don't be – your attractiveness, according to research, shows that no matter how good looking you are, it won't have an effect on whether you're convicted or acquitted. (See References, p. 256.) And these studies go back as far as forty years.

> Attractiveness was predictive of both minimum and maximum sentences – the more attractive the defendant, the less severe the sentence imposed.

And what if I told you this bias wasn't just based on attraction, but on how 'baby-faced' they were? 'The more baby-faced an adult was, the less likely he/she was found to be guilty for "intentional actions" in civil claims.' (See References, p. 256.)

If you look at the back of this book, you'll see me smiling – and yes, my teeth are veneers. In fact, I don't even have my own front two teeth any more. Growing up, for some strange reason, I never liked metal touching my teeth. So, even though I had serious overcrowding, I never wanted braces – the idea of them made me feel sick. By twenty-three, though, I was a bit fed up with my teeth being so crooked (sometimes in rugby I wouldn't wear a mouthguard, as I thought at least if I knocked them out I'd have to deal with them). Well, one day I went to see my dentist about getting something done.

The dentist said he could remove my two front teeth and create a 'bridge' across the front; it would mean a few weeks with temporary teeth and then a straight smile. I agreed, signed up on a payment plan and went from very crooked teeth to immaculately straight ones. When asked why I did it, it was actually to do with my job at the time. I was working in recruitment and some of the clients were fairly large household names. I thought that no matter how nice my suit, my shoes or my tie, if I had poor teeth people would immediately discredit me based on them. And I later found out that the science behind this thinking shows it to be true (see References, p. 256):

One's attractiveness does impinge on achievement and psychological well-being.

Our brains will automatically (System 1 – remember?) draw a bias, a prejudice and a level of trust in a person based just on their looks, how they dress and how they present themselves. It is human nature, after all. Have you noticed that when people are asked what they look for in a partner they often say 'nice teeth'. To them, it's something they hold in high regard. (I personally think that it can be a subtle hint to another person about their oral hygiene because, let's face it, no one likes bad breath.) My old man (that means dad in English) has always said that whenever he met someone, he'd look at their shoes, then their tie, how it was done up. This, for him, would be a visual representation of that person's professionalism, attention to detail and perhaps self-admin.

When people do the same with teeth it's their System 1 drawing conclusions about someone else's standards of hygiene. I'd hypothesize that perhaps if someone takes good care of those things, you could rely on them to bring the same traits to a relationship, bringing up a family and life in general.

The aforementioned biases are very real – they are a part of being human, and a better understanding of them is integral to us to developing socially and economically. Just as we must not come to conclusions in science without evidence, we cannot draw conclusions about someone based on just their appearance. We're no longer apes in the jungle and we need to act more like it. Having my teeth 'done' was probably one of the best decisions I've made. In a world where people judge very quickly, even a few seconds on social media is the difference between someone deciding they want to listen or they want to move on. I'm not advocating that everyone should have perfect teeth* or jump to get veneers, but it's important to know that your appearance is a big factor in other people's subconscious bias.

* If you're 50/50 about having work done to your teeth I will semi-hypocritically tell you not to. I feel that we all have our unique 'looks' and sometimes I feel my teeth are too perfect. It sounds crazy, yes, I know, but I can't help but feel we're made up of imperfections and that's what makes us human.

Why?

People don't buy what you do, they buy why you do it.

Simon Sinek, *Start with Why: How Great Leaders Inspire
Everyone to Take Action*

'Why' we do things is at the root of the most powerful emotion when it comes to human behaviour in my opinion. We do crazy and unimaginable things not based on what, not based on how but based on why. For instance, patriotism: soldiers who go to war, wear the badge of their nation and go to war for the cause. That's not a what, that's a why. Their why is about love for their country; their why is ingrained deeper than their salary and their position. When people are willing to die for a cause, it's because of why, not what.

This book is more about why I wrote it than what I write, or even how I write it. Over the years, I have had countless criticisms of my approach and one of my favourite ways to disarm someone is to ask them, 'Why do you think I am saying this?' 'What do you think my motive is for doing this?' When people can understand WHY I am doing something, they can then overlook how I do it or even what I am doing. I like to think that those who like me – those who buy my books, read my posts or listen to my podcasts – do so because of why I do what I do, not what I do.

If you came to me with a business idea, I would not ask you what you're doing, I wouldn't ask how you're going to do it, I would simply ask why you're doing it. If you can't answer that, I'd heavily suggest you didn't do it in the first place.

I've been doing pretty much the same thing now for years, and recently I have experienced an element of so-called 'fame', incredible payslips and opportunities I never dreamed of. But that's not why I do what I do. The way you can know that for sure is because I did this for years without any of that and I still loved every minute of it.

Over time, and as my following has grown, my 'how' has changed, my 'what' has changed **but my 'why' has never changed**. Speaking to a crowd of 10 or 10,000, the reason why I do something is not influenced, nor will it be, and no one can take away my 'why' either. This is what makes it so powerful.

'Why do you do what you do, James?'

Most days I'm asked if it gets boring answering the same questions each day. No, it doesn't. Why? Because I know that the person asking isn't asking for the sake of it. With every sentence I am instilling information in the mind of someone who needs it and perhaps also the mind of someone else who is watching or listening. There is a butterfly effect in life with each and every life form on the planet. For me to give mere minutes of my time to change the course of a few hundred for the better is not something I'd take lightly. Upskilling, empowering and educating hundreds is one thing, but the compounding interest of that through a recurring daily habit is powerful. That reaches lives, passes down through generations, and I'd like to think 'my why' is a ripple of information, attitude and approach that can continue throughout the years after I'm gone. That isn't just limited to me. Any single person on the planet with a strong enough 'why' can do the exact same thing. You can, but only if you choose to.

I also think I could be the person for someone else that I once needed, and that's powerful, too. I think to myself each day how my life could have been different if I'd had someone to listen to, learn from, and develop from, and I don't take that for granted.

Intrinsic vs extrinsic motivators

What and how don't fuel the daily fires in us. They just don't. Author and motivational speaker Simon Sinek has done a fantastic job over the years explaining how Apple have excelled beyond their competitors because they are 'why' driven; even in their adverts they don't explain what they are releasing but *why* they are releasing it. And when we look at motivators for people's 'why' we can see intrinsic and extrinsic motivators.

Extrinsic motivation is when you engage in behaviour in order to get something in return or even to avoid something unpleasant, but not because you like doing it or find it satisfying. For instance, if you do something purely for the money it's extrinsically motivated.

Intrinsic motivation is when you engage in behaviour because it's personally rewarding. The behaviour in itself is its own reward.

So, if your mum says she's going to lose her shit if you don't make your bed, you make it to avoid punishment (extrinsic); however, if you're like me and you walk into your room at night and see the bed perfectly made and take pleasure in pulling back the corner to get back into it, that's intrinsic motivation.

I can often get caught up in the wrong reward system when I go for a run. Sometimes I get too involved in the time of the run, beating a personal best and posting it on my social media. Instead, I should just enjoy the run, the audiobook that I listen to and the fact I can hit my daily step count while exercising.

When people are told to run for fat loss or because their doctor told them to, they're doing it for extrinsic motivation, to avoid something unpleasant, such as illnesses associated with obesity like Type II diabetes. If you were to decide who would still be running this time next year out of Jack (who was told to run by his doctor – extrinsic) or Bill (who just loves running – intrinsic), it's clear that it's much more likely to be the person who is intrinsically motivated.

Extrinsic motivation has its place too, though. Without it we would never clean up after ourselves, go to work or do things we may not want to do. Offering a reward (extrinsic) for doing an intrinsically motivated task can decrease motivation. This is known as the 'overjustification effect'. Let' say you have a child who is playing with a puzzle and you reward them with sweets for doing it, you'll soon realize that when you remove the sweets the child's drive for doing the puzzle will diminish. So, it's a good idea to identify how you're motivated with tasks to ensure that you don't ever undermine your intrinsic motivation to do it in the first place.

Have you ever noticed that adults often don't invest their time in the right places – for instance, self-help books that would almost definitely benefit their personal or career development? Throughout our time in education we're constantly told we 'have to' read certain things or that we 'must' study certain topics. Perhaps this confuses people, because the motivation for these tasks becomes extrinsic rather than intrinsic. This is ironic because that feeling is stunting our growth and certainly holding us back from our full potential in life. The solution? We need to adjust our thinking to pursue intrinsic hobbies and activities that benefit and enrich our quality of life, our finite time on this spinning rock. This links back to adjusting our mindset, our approach, flipping our existing bias on its head.

Why is what keeps us going. **Why** is what drives us forward with a task. It's not what we do, but **why** we do it; not how we do it, but **why**.

Whether it's weight loss, running a business or asking someone out on a date, it all breaks down to **why**. If you keep your **why** in your mind, on your wall or saved as a background on your phone or laptop, it will drive you much further than merely a reminder of what you are doing.

TASK

Remember, you don't need to be motivated – you need to ensure you don't demotivate yourself when you're on the road to accomplishing something. Rather than putting some clichéd quote somewhere like 'believe in yourself', why not put your why on the wall? Think about it in detail and don't lie. For years, I had clients lie to me about their why. They'd tell me 'I want to get fit' or 'I want to be healthier', and I would always question them, telling them to stop saying what they thought I wanted to hear and to just tell me their *real* why. And the real why would usually be to do with something much deeper: fucking with the lights on, their partner being the one who instigates sex for once, the confidence to stand up in their line of work or even to walk away from a relationship that has gone stale. My why right now is ensuring that other people don't go down the path I was led down. So, think about yours. Think deep. Write it down. And make it real.

Making it Real

Thoughts exist, to us anyway. Ideas, concepts, goals or dreams are likely to slip away from us, so we must write them down. We are so confident in our ability to remember our ideas – until we forget them. Whenever an idea crosses your mind make it real. I use the notes section on my phone. Just writing it down locks it that bit tighter into my memory. Ideas never come when we need them. Perhaps we can blame systems 1 and 2 for that (see p. 138). But blaming won't get us anywhere. I am so grateful that modern smartphones are waterproof because I often reach out of the shower to scribble down ideas that come to me as I stand under the warm water. Content ideas, book chapters, podcast debates – I make a note and later, as I cast an eye back over them, I realize how grateful I am that I wrote them down.

A self-set goal, however random, is made so much more tangible if it is written or typed – on a whiteboard, a chalk board, in a notes section or as a saved background, there to remind us. We can't overlook the simple fact that reminding ourselves is a powerful tool. I once saw a study that changed my mind about religion altogether. Students in a class were asked to perform a maths test, to mark it, then shred it. They then told the supervisor how many questions they got correct and were awarded a dollar for each one. Unbeknown to the quiz takers the shredding machine was fake and their tests were totalled against the dollars given. It turned out that there was a fair bit of dishonesty among the students. The experiment was then repeated with different participants, and this time they were given tokens instead of dollars and the tokens could be redeemed for dollars down the hall. What happened? The rate of dishonesty increased, meaning more dollars were claimed via tokens. A third group of students was lined up, but before taking the test they were asked to recite as many of the Ten Commandments as they could remember. They then went on to perform the test and were the least dishonest group when it came to reporting their results, suggesting a link between ingraining someone with morals or ethics before a task and increasing their honesty and integrity. That day, I remember removing my atheist status. I decided to no longer try to convert people to my belief of no beliefs and instead to let people decide what they believe as their prerogative. Why? Because whatever someone uses to keep them on track is up to them; it's about making it real.

> **TASK**
>
> Think about something you want to do, think about why, then think about how you can make it real. Print it, write it, save it.

For me, one of the most important 'make it real' tools was a vision board on my wall. To my left, as I turned the light on, it was right there. So, no matter how cold or dark it was or how tired I felt, I would have a reminder of why I was waking up and what for. It would be like an electric pulse through the body and as I would shower, I would be mindful of what I needed to accomplish that day.

Newton's Laws

Sir Isaac Newton was a top bloke. I'll explain why. So, in the seventeenth century an apple supposedly fell from a tree and hit him on the head. I'm not sure if that is completely true, but from there Isaac came up with the 'law of gravity'. I love to remind people that he didn't invent gravity, he just noted its existence. Imagine how many people had lived on Earth until then, fully unaware of the force that was pulling them to the very ground they walked on. That's why I love to challenge people on their thoughts and perceptions in daily life and even in relationships; you don't have to be aware of a force for it to act upon you every second of every day.

Gravity is not unique to Earth. It's everywhere in the universe, and the larger something is, the more gravity it has. About twenty years after Newton discovered gravity, he presented his three laws of motion:

- ▸ The first law states that if an object is at rest with no force on it, it will remain at rest. This is known as inertia. Basically, to remain unchanged.
- ▸ The second law states that the velocity of an object changes when it is subjected to an external force. This is where the complex maths of force, mass and acceleration come into play, but this isn't 'Not a Physics Book', so I'll move on …
- ▸ The third law states that for every action there is an equal and opposite reaction.

The third law is the most important because it is applicable to every aspect of life as we know it. If there is an equal and opposite reaction for every action, we must therefore be confident in understanding and believing in the choices we make. Protecting our energy is so important because when we engage in things that drain us it does make a huge difference.

Energy cannot be created or destroyed, it can only be changed from one form to another.

Albert Einstein

Life around us, relationships or a car driving past are all forms of energy passing from one to another – from the inertia of the car slowing down, the fuel that causes locomotion and the exhaust fumes coming out, to the hand turning this page, using energy from your last meal.

The point of this science lesson is to teach you that energy is always moving and you must protect your own. You only get so much in a lifetime. So, if your ex wants to argue, don't get involved; if someone wants to wind you up, don't give it the energy. If you choose to (and again, it is a choice), you will be giving up energy that you could instead be giving to those you love, the business or profession in which you work or at least to something that would give you a much better return on energy expended.

- ▶ Use Newton's first law to ask someone for their number or for a job promotion; if you don't act upon an object, it will stay where it is.
- ▶ Use the second law to give more force and effort to those areas where you wish to see change. The more you apply, the faster you can go.

► Use the third law to ensure that your reaction benefits the energy equation; don't let people steal your energy. It's changing form at all times, so make sure you're investing yours in the right place that benefits you. More often than not, arguing and negativity are just a waste of energy that could be put to better use.

~~Not~~ the Final Chapter

What if I told you that there is a version of you that lives in the future after reading this book? Let's call it your 'future self', and your future self is one impressive fucking person. They walk the walk, they talk the talk, and holy shit, your friends and family see your future self as a brand new person. You wear the same clothes, but you wear them differently. You have the same voice, but you sound a little different. You have more gravitas and you're more sure of every string of words you put together. You no longer take shit from people around you and you're hellbent on accomplishing what you desire, not what others think you desire. Your future self is … quite frankly fucking impressive.

Right now, as you read this chapter, there are things out of your control. There's physics – gravity keeping you in your chair (or risking you falling over if you're standing up listening to this on a busy train). Then there's biology – as your cells regenerate, oxygen goes in and carbon dioxide out in a gaseous exchange. There's thermodynamics at play when you exercise and when you select what to eat for your next meal. There's hydrodynamics at play when next you swim in the sea or a lake. They will continue to exist no matter what you do, long after you've read these final pages, so by all means eat well, be active, sleep enough each night and remain hydrated. But there is chemistry I hope to have influenced at least. Maybe to feel some goosebumps as you read this final chapter, as I am while writing it.

But that isn't the point of this book, is it? In fact, it's very far from it.

The changes from the turn of these final pages cannot be measured, they cannot be weighed and they cannot be put under a microscope for examination. **Audacity, tenacity, grit, willpower, confidence, resilience, ambition and a willingness to put yourself in uncomfortable conversations and situations are not quantifiable by mere numbers or metrics, not even by science as we know it.** So many elements in your life from the initial chapter will remain the same, but so many need to change as you put this book down for perhaps the last time (maybe revisiting certain topics when you need to).

You need to sit back and think about what you want from your time on this spinning rock and what is important to you – not to anyone else, but you. Don't compare your values to others'; don't be influenced by your parents or the societal norms, as this is unique to you and you alone. You don't go through life to make other people happy; you do it to make yourself happy. A successful relationship is two people sharing their own happiness with each other, not one having to provide it for both. Whether you want a simple life, a complex life, a busy life or a quiet one, you must decide and then construct it as you wish.

Real success and real wealth are subjective, based upon your feelings, your tastes and your opinions. Life is not destination based, it's journey based; it's all about the ride, not the final stop. And to see wealth, freedom or success objectively as a fixed amount or a finite sum will not grant you an enjoyable journey. Don't expect a certain amount of money to make you happy, because you may attain it and realize nothing has changed.

With a new mindset you can realize someone having more money does not make them richer, someone with more material objects is not certain to be happier. It's time to break down your future anxieties, time to dismantle your thoughts of uncertainty and to stop a constant worry about the future ahead. **Your future self has your back, and you need to put faith in that.**

It's time to take risks and I know you're scared of what is to come if you take my advice. But I want you to act and do what is necessary for today; tomorrow is another today, after all.

Your values are of most importance: what you prioritize and what you don't. What truly makes you happy? What do you really want to get from life? This is as unique as your DNA, so don't look left or right to anyone else for the answers. Asking someone else for what should make you happy could be like asking a blind person for directions.

Be bold, take risks and leave the 'blueprint to life' behind. Leave it to those who are happy to follow it. If it was right for you, you wouldn't have made it this far – you would have rejected my notions sooner and stopped turning the pages. The reason you're here is because you're climbing a ladder, just like everyone else. However, you're coming to realize, bit by bit, that it's probably not the right ladder for you. You're looking around and not seeing anyone else questioning it, and there-fore thinking you're broken in some way. So, it's important to remind yourself constantly that it's better to be halfway up the correct ladder than it is to be at the very top of the wrong one.

Those worries that are weeks, months, years ahead? Future you has them covered. Any problems, hiccups or tough situations, I am sure your future self can get you out of, no problem. Ask yourself this: have you ever let yourself down thus far in life? **Adversity breeds your best performances.** Never doubt the version of yourself in the future because it's a hardened and more robust version of the person you are today. Be confident in the person you are going to be. Cherish the adversity ahead as your biggest growth will come from it.

There is a fabric to your identity, a fabric to your mind, and it has no limits to how it is stretched. There are no stupid human beings, I refuse

251

to believe that. We merely have fully utilized and non-utilized mindsets. We have those people who exponentially stretch the fabric of their minds and those who don't, who believe they're limited. You must stretch your mind's fabric at every opportunity possible; you must do it to prove to yourself that you're not limited in anything you do. We are not born confident, we are not born with skills, we are not born 'naturally good' at anything. Any limits in your mind are self-imposed; you have created them, you have believed them, you have allowed them to be barriers to your own success, but they hold no weight, and you can dismantle them just as fast as you created them, if you choose to.

Don't leave anything for the latter end of your life because, quite frankly you don't know how long you'll be around for. All the things you're waiting to do in life can be done now, so why not do them? Better to retire having nothing left to accomplish than to hope you'll have the energy to do it at sixty-five. Hedging your bets on a ticket for a way out is about as futile as hedging your bets that you'll make it to an older age with a perfect bill of health or without responsibilities to those around you.

Stop spending your days worrying about your CV and fiddling the dates around in a bid to impress people you've never even met. There are so many people not living their lives or doing what they want because they're worried about how a stranger will perceive a piece of paper with their name, a few jobs and the words 'Curriculum Vitae' at the top, and I'm here to point out that worrying about that is moronic. Live your life the way you want and if someone can't handle the fact that you took a few big breaks out of life to fucking live it, then perhaps you're applying for a work environment that isn't the right fit for you.

Any relative success will bring you the feeling of being an imposter. Get used to it and trust me, it's not going away any time soon. Don't be afraid of things going wrong because it's where we learn the most.

Success doesn't come without lessons learned along the way, so don't see mistakes as bad things, merely adjustments to the course. Your future self won't be half the fucking hero they are going to be without the mistakes that are coming, so look forward to and cherish each and every one and ride them out when they come.

Becoming your future self is better than _being_ your future self. Enjoy every step of the journey and especially the tough days. The good isn't the good without the bad, after all. One thing I need to tell you is that not everyone around you is coming with you on this journey to the person you're going to be. It will, for most of you, be a time to make cuts, and I don't need to point fingers because you already know deep down. I know you do. Throughout this book you will have got a feeling for who will be coming with you and who, unfortunately, will be left behind.

I can't do this for you. I can't. I've done all I can between the first page and this one. I have pulled back the string on the bow with you through these chapters and you need to decide whether you fire _or if you don't_.

We only really make sense of our existence on the planet in what we call 'our life so far' when we look backwards and connect the dots, each one unique and making total sense in retrospect. However, it's time to put into practice what I have taught you to determine where those future dots are going to lie.

I'm not your life coach. I'm not your motivational guru. But I know that if you put these words into practice I will have changed your life. The day you look back on where everything changed for you is not far off from right now. Take a deep breath, think of your first course of action, write it down, make it real and begin to plan out how to make it happen. My last piece of advice is crucial, imperative, vital and can't be forgotten, and that is:

Don't forget to fucking enjoy it – something that is so often over-looked, so often drowned by worries, so often lost from our minds during each moment of each day. Ultimately, if you do one thing, remember to enjoy the fucking ride.

And I'll leave you with the best advice my dad has ever given me throughout my life whenever I've asked him, 'Why?' – whether I should do something that I wasn't sure about.

I'll never forget what he has told me every single time:

Well, why not? You're a long time dead, son.

Geoffrey Smith

James

References

p. 8 https://psycnet.apa.org/record/2015-16536-003

p. 9 https://www.ncbi.nlm.nih.gov/pmc/articles/PMC3678674/

p. 12 https://www.pnas.org/content/107/38/16489#ref-21

p. 12 Quoidbach, J., Dunn, E. W., Petrides, K. V., Mikolajczak, M. (2010), 'Money Giveth, Money Taketh Away: The Dual Effect of Wealth on Happiness', *Psychological Science*, 21:759–763.

p. 32 Dweck C. S., 'Mindsets and Malleable Minds: Implications for Giftedness and Talent', in: Subotnik R. F., Robinson A., Callahan, C. M., Gubbins, E. J. (eds), 'Malleable Minds: Translating Insights from Psychology and Neuroscience to Gifted Education', National Research Center on the Gifted and Talented, University of Connecticut; Storrs, CT, USA: 2012. pp. 7–18.

p. 44 Granberg, Donald & Brown, Thad, A. (1995), 'The Monty Hall Dilemma', *Personality and Social Psychology Bulletin*, 21 (7): 711–729

p. 51 https://www.lottery.co.uk/lotto/odds

p. 78 https://bigthink.com/politics-current-affairs/how-finlands-education-system-works?rebelltitem=1#rebelltitem1

p. 83 Tordjman, S., Chokron, S., Delorme, R., Charrier, A., Bellissant, E., Jaafari, N. and Fougerou, C., 'Melatonin: Pharmacology, Functions and Therapeutic Benefits', *Current Neuropharmacology*, April 2017, 15 (3), pp.434–43: https://www.ncbi.nlm.nih.gov/pmc/articles/PMC5405617/

p. 84 National Sleep Foundation Sleep and Teens Task Force, 'Adolescent Sleep Needs and Patterns: Research Report and Resource Guide', Washington: National Sleep Foundation; 2000. pp. 1–26.

p. 84 Gangwisch, J. E., Babiss, L.A., Malaspina, D., et al., 'Earlier parental set bedtimes as a protective factor against depression and suicidal ideation', *Sleep*, 2010;33(1):97–106.

p. 98 https://pubmed.ncbi.nlm.nih.gov/29116983/

p. 115 Khaw et al., 2008; Ford et al., 2011 (https://www.ncbi.nlm.nih.gov/pmc/articles/PMC4468355/)

p. 119 https://en.wikipedia.org/wiki/Confidence

p. 121 Hewitt, John P. (2009), *Oxford Handbook of Positive Psychology*, Oxford University Press, pp. 217–24

p. 122 https://www.sciencedirect.com/science/article/abs/pii/S0191886902000788

p. 139 Which line is longer? The Müller-Lyer illusion (Müller-Lyer, 1889). Knowing that the two lines are of equal length does not stop them appearing of different lengths.

p. 146 http://bora.uib.no/bitstream/handle/1956/15969/Final-draft-Tine-og-Sarah.pdf?sequence=1

p. 146 https://www.ncbi.nlm.nih.gov/pubmed/26132913

p. 161 https://www.gov.uk/government/publications/health-profile-for-england/chapter-2-major-causes-of-death-and-how-they-have-changed

p. 175 nasa.gov

p. 196 Neil DeGrass Tyson's Twitter @neiltyson

p. 214 https://en.wikipedia.org/wiki/Regression_toward_the_mean

p. 223 https://www.ncbi.nlm.nih.gov/pubmed/14768844

p. 225 Jones, 1995; Craft, Magyar, Becker, & Fetlz, 2003; Woodman & Hardy, 2003

p. 225 https://en.wikiversity.org/wiki/Motivation_and_emotion/Book/2018/Arousal_and_sporting_performance

p. 234 Stewart, John E., 'Defendant's Attractiveness as a Factor in the Outcome of Criminal Trials: An Observational Study' (1980); https://www.researchgate.net/publication/229629159_Defendant%27s_Attractiveness_as_a_Factor_in_the_Outcome_of_Criminal_Trials_An_Observational_Study1

p. 234 https://www.thelawproject.com.au/insights/attractiveness-bias-in-the-legal-system

p. 234 https://psycnet.apa.org/record/1992-14970-001

p. 235 https://www.researchgate.net/publication/271808429_The_Impact_of_Physical_Attractiveness_on_Achievement_and_Psychological_Well-Being

Acknowledgements

My James Smith Academy members, your trust and belief in what I do has given me the freedom and the time to pursue things I enjoy, just like writing this book, and future books to come.

James Shaw, should I say 'brethren'? Thanks for the years of support and passive-aggressive messages to give me a kick in the arse.

Pippa, thanks for my first ever plug on social media and being there at every turn for me.

Andrew and the rest of my James Smith Academy coaches for supporting the team and me daily.

Big special thank you to every member, follower, subscriber, recipient, liker, watcher, double tapper and sharer that's existed past and present.

LT Summers, Dizza, J. Alexander, Fezley Snipes, Lord of the Mic, Sven Gudvunsen, Cammatron and the Willey. See you on the Book Tour <3

James

Index

259

THE INSPIRATIONAL
#1 *SUNDAY TIMES* BESTSELLER

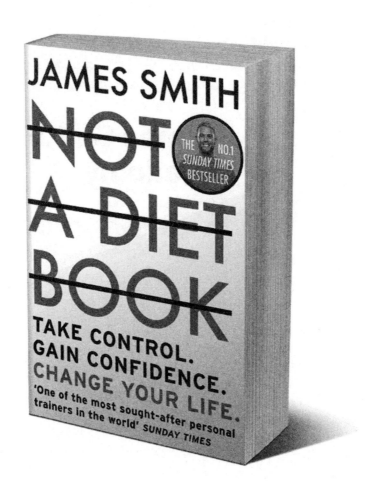

OUT NOW

If you enjoyed the book and would like to see more of what
I can do to help you in the next stage of your journey,
feel free to head to the James Smith Academy:

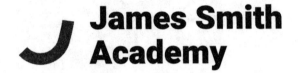

www.jamessmithacademy.com
@Jamessmithpt

'It's time to take risks.

Your future self has your back, you need to put faith in that. Be confident in that person you are going to be. Relish the adversity ahead, as your biggest growth will come from it.'